TAPAS LIFE

A rich and rewarding life
after your long career

BY ANDREW ROBIN

Dedicated to my fine family

My gratitude goes to Paula, Cynthia, Marli, and José; and to those who gave me feedback along the way

CONTENTS

INTRODUCTION

You could be retired for decades — so
you might as well get good at it!

I f you get to 65, with some care you're likely to live another 20 to 25 years or more. This book can help you
get good at living those years well. And it's *different*
from other "retirement" books. I call it *Tapas Life* because,
like the small dishes of Spain that make up a tasty meal,
having a variety of activities and ways of being that are
all to my liking make for a rich and rewarding life. Since
I've found this excellent life, which is such a complement
to my years raising a family as primary breadwinner, I've
written this book to share how you can get your own
Tapas Life.

**Think of it as a *how-to* book intended to be useful
to you.** I hope it will facilitate your journey into what I
call a post–"Long Career" life you love, rather than the

undesirable gradual decline experienced by many who retire.

When I say "Long Career," I'm referring to the several decades that most folks have spent working for a living. I'm 68 and I've met a lot of them — many of whom seem lost in terms of knowing or being able to plan what kind of life lies ahead for them.

Sure, many of us say we're looking forward to travel, reading, outdoor activities, and such. And that might seem like heaven, especially if your mental model is School > Work/Family > some Golden Years > Game Over.

But too many people I meet haven't come to terms with the fact that while those heavenly activities will be terrific for 6 or 12 or 18 months, it's highly unlikely they'll be enough to keep life rich and rewarding for two to three decades. In fact, one fellow I interviewed said, "It's hard to wrap my head around doing this for another 25 years."

Our increased longevity has certainly been written and talked about a lot. Yet people I know in the 55-to-70 range have seemingly let the notion that their third phase of life may be just as long or longer than the Long Career portion of their life roll right off their back. And I've seen precious little thought given to those extra years, except perhaps on the dollars-and-cents front.

Let's look at the facts. Most men I ask think their life expectancy is 77 or 78, "per the mortality tables." Well, they're right about the tables, but the actual number in the U.S. is 76.1 *from birth*. On the other hand, if you actually make it to age 65, then your new life expectancy shoots up to 83.1. (After all, young people, especially boys/men under 25, are likelier to die prematurely as a result of car wrecks, gangs, wars, drugs, and general mischief.) Once you hit 65, if you're in decent good health, eat reasonably well, do some exercise, and aren't cursed with bad genes, it's pretty likely you'll live into your late 80s or beyond. The same stats for women are 81.1 from birth, 85.6 if you make it to 65, and well into your 90s if you manage to stay relatively fit. Those numbers are even higher for people in a higher socio-economic stratum who tend to eat well, be well educated, exercise, are less apt to smoke, have more opportunity to challenge their mind, have access to excellent medical help, and are less likely to be exposed to potentially life-shortening environments. Women born in the wealthy, tiny municipality of Monaco, for instance, have a life expectancy of 93 at birth!

The simple fact is that life expectancy at 65 has grown 20 times faster over the past 50 years than over the preceding century. When I look at the IRS's Required Minimum Distributions table for IRAs, it's telling me that at 66, my RMD implies I'll live to 97. If I get to 80, the table implies 99. And if I get to 90, the IRS wants me to do RMDs such that I'll finish distributing my IRA savings at 101. The IRS has stated that they don't want to see IRAs used as estate-planning vehicles (and recently the tax laws were changed accordingly), but rather that one should use their last IRA distribution just as they die. While their numbers are more optimistic than insurance mortality tables (I guess they don't want people running out of their IRA money), it's a reminder that with a little luck and care, most of us will likely be around longer than we think.

So, yeah, another 20 to 30 years after your Long Career is complete.

It would be great if everyone knew this, because recognizing the reality is a necessary precursor to adapting to it and making it work for you.

MJ Elmore, an investor and philanthropist, noted that she had "thought wrong about longevity." She once thought that after so-called retirement age, life would gradually wind down. Now, in her mid-60s, she realizes she's actually in her "third trimester of life."

Consider this book your road map to that third trimester — a very particular kind of road map. Instead of seeing people retire and be lost, bored, and possibly depressed, my aim is to see people live an interesting, varied, and fulfilling life after their Long Career. What follows is a step-by-step approach that will give you a fresh opportunity to *really engage* with the decades ahead. It's filled with my personal experiences and a couple of dozen conversations with other "retirees," all designed to lead you into the rich and rewarding life you deserve. Enjoy.

• • •

CHAPTER ONE

MY OWN TAPAS LIFE

In one kiss, you'll know all I haven't said.

— Pablo Neruda,
  Nobel Prize–winning
  Chilean poet

W e've all heard a lot about bucket lists, which usually consist of all of our dreams and can't-miss adventures packed into one, big overwhelming…bucket. That's all well and good, but I believe you can create a plan that's more creative, flexible, and personalized than a mere bucket list, more wide-ranging than simply pursuing a particular passion, and more effective than simply going with the flow. I call this plan a Tapas Life because I liken it to eating a variety of tasty small plates instead of one or two run-of-the-mill entrées that happen to be the most popular on the menu. *Tapas,* as you may know, are the little dishes served in Spain. A few shrimp with garlic (*Gambas al Ajillo*), a potato quiche (*Tortilla Española*), some olives, some cheese, and so on. Rather than eat one big dish, you sample from a few little dishes to start, and then another and another until you're satisfied. When my wife and I traveled in Spain (for a vacation and to visit our son during his college semester abroad), we enjoyed tapas galore. It's such a great way to enjoy food — and life.

I haven't always eaten — or worked — like that. Often, during my Long Career, it seemed to me that life was like one *big* dish: a combo of family and job that was all-consuming, crowding over the edges of the plate. Instead of delicate tapas, with lots of anticipation between courses, my life was more like "The Big Texan," the 72-ounce porterhouse steak served by a restaurant in Texas I frequented (and believe me, after The Big Texan, there was not much room for anything else!). Suffice it to say that if you ate the whole thing in one sitting — and survived — they'd give it to you for free.…

By contrast, with tapas, you can have some of this, some of that, and some of the other things, too — in other words, more variety. If you don't like one, you can set it aside and get something different. Or take a pause from eating all together.

Such is the nature of the Tapas Life: You can assemble a set of activities and ways of being that nourish you and add up to the customized life you want. And you can always add, remove, or change out any Tapa(s) along the way. *Because you're the chef and the eater.*

I guess you could call me a tapas kind of guy. Over the years, I've taken different approaches to living my life. This may be because I grew up in two different countries — the U.S. and Mexico — which made it easier for me to see, early on, that there are multiple ways to live life. In the U.S., life seems to be more harried, and in Mexico, more laid back. There's more focus on the individual in the U.S., and more focus on family in Mexico. There's more money and there are more jobs in the U.S. than in Mexico, and economic matters get more attention. And of course, foods and culture are quite different. I like both, and they helped me see that different paths are possible.

One of my first swerves from the straight and narrow happened when I was 19 and dropped out of a famous university after only a year. The teaching was so very awful that it seemed like a waste of tuition (they kept telling me it would get better my junior and senior years — a pretty poor way to run a prestigious university, IMHO). It was the early '70s, and I went home and started a computer business with my father, who was retired and bored to tears. He knew the business end and I took quickly to the technical end, learning programming and computer repair when those things were largely unknown; we ended up bringing each other along for five years, until I figured it was time to get a college degree. In retrospect, it was a great experience doing tech in those early days — yet another nudge for me in the direction of a different sort of life.

After going back to school at another university, where the teaching was (happily) much better, I finished, then went on to get an MBA from a well-known eastern business school. This unusual path was a good one for me because when I did go back to school, I knew more about myself, more about wanting to work in tech, and more about what sorts of geographies/climates suited me. I was also simply more mature and knew what I wanted to learn. In retrospect, I suppose it's useful for many 18-year-olds to head off to college, especially for socialization and to learn independence, but how on earth can we expect them to know what they want to major in and what their interests are when they've only lived in the home cocoon? (I believe that's why only about a quarter of people wind up in a career that matches what they majored in.)

After B-school, I decided I wanted to live someplace warm and to work in something related to computers but not *in* computers (frankly, by that time, I was bored with computers). I got a job in microchips and advanced well in that field, eventually getting a good offer that led me to Silicon Valley in the early years. When I arrived there, I looked up my now-wife's parents, who I knew had retired in the area. Coincidentally, her family and mine both moved from Chicago to Mexico City when we were kids to grab an entrepreneurial opportunity, and we kids met and became friends in a big group in middle school. When I learned that she was in the area, too, I called her up to get together. A few months later, on New Year's Eve, we got engaged.

Before getting married in '85, my now-wife and I talked a lot about what we wanted out of life. Both of us wanted to pursue our careers, and we were both doing very well (I was soon to be promoted to Director of Marketing of a significant company; she was Sales/Marketing Manager of the 13 western states for an industrial automation company). What was more unusual is that both of us said we wanted a turn serving as the primary at-home caregiver to the children we would have one day. And we did just that: My wife quit her job to start a family, and she had the kids from birth until middle school or so, while I continued working. Then, when the kids were 13 and 15, I left my job as VP of Marketing to become a housedad, and my wife launched a new work life. The timing was good because she had just finished her Ph.D., and I was quite done with corporate life and ready for more time with the kids. Carole became a partner in organization development consulting and then a Lecturer at Stanford Business School. She's now co-founder of a nonprofit seeking to change the culture in Silicon Valley, and also an executive coach. Not exactly the path everyone takes — yet it was a good one for us.

Except that after our youngest went off to college, I found myself with a lot more time on my hands and no agenda, no plans. I felt a little adrift. So I contemplated for a while, just sitting with where I was (as an introvert, that's my process). And then I started taking action: trying something, then something else, simply seeking to move forward. I felt no need to find a whole new job, and certainly not any need to prove anything to anyone. I just had to get moving. There was no real method to my tapas-like samplings — my new life and activities were simply emergent and sort of accumulated.

That may sound haphazard, but it led over the next four years to the gradual assembly of a life I love. When a friend stopped me on the street one day and asked what I was up to, I told him I was "**living my Tapas Life.**" The concept just rolled out of my mouth like a gumball.

I've written about myself here so you can see that I've been willing to try approaches that others might not. That's relevant, because what I'm going to describe in *Tapas Life* is a *different* approach from those usually put forth in mainstream "retirement" books. I write about myself to help you see that there are many possibilities available to you.

As wonderful as the Tapas Life has been for me, it surely isn't for everyone. Some people are just fine living a life of leisure until they fade away. Others prefer to work until they're carried out of the office with their boots on (à la Warren Buffett). There are also those who, after their Long Career, will start in on a second "Big Texan," and then a third. All good, all good.

But if those options don't feel satisfying to you, this book offers another buy: putting together a self-curated new life born of an array of possibilities. When you read this book, you'll learn how to assemble your very own Tapas Life, step by step. And you

may well also come to know yourself better as a result of the process.

One more thing of note. In his book _Man's Search for Meaning_, Holocaust survivor Viktor Frankl writes, "Everything can be taken from a [person] but one thing: the last of the human freedoms — to choose one's attitude in any given set of circumstances, to choose one's own way." You've got a lot of _choice_ available to you for the taking, and it's vital to envision and choose a life-filled, energetic, useful, meaningful path. To get started, try this exercise:

Exercise: Write out a list of choices available to you as you contemplate and embark on your next several decades of a rich and rewarding life. Hint: It should be a _loooooooooong_ list! Kick it around with people close to you. Examples abound as the book unfolds. **Paraphrasing the Neruda quote at the top of the chapter, Taste one Tapa and you'll start to know all you haven't seen!**

CHAPTER TWO

• • •

WHITE RABBIT IN A SNOWSTORM

I don't think that scheduling is uncreative. I think that structure is required for creativity.

— Twyla Tharp,
American choreographer and dancer

When my wife and I swapped roles, she immediately skipped town to a gig in Australia for three weeks. She had agreed to become partner in a small consulting firm that did a lot of work for a big company over there, and that was her first assignment. Me, I went through baptism by fire in the full-time care and feeding of teens. The truth is that I was very lucky — I had my work cut out for me.

That's not true for most people. After the goodbye lunch with colleagues, the following Monday, Tuesday, or Wednesday may bring the slightly shocking realization that they're no longer due back at work. After a few weeks or months, it might sink in that they're not even on vacation. Nope, they're not actually going back to that job this week or next week, or any week, for that matter.

One person I interviewed noted that "this is different — rather than work being added, it was *subtracted*." Another said that friends had cautioned him about "the scary freefall into retirement." To avoid that, he told himself he'd do many things he hadn't had time for, fill his time wisely, avoid making rash decisions, and allow himself to ease into it.

To my unscientific eye, the most extreme case of the "scary freefall" happens with people in the medical profession. After decades of having virtually every minute of their lives scheduled, they face calendars that are now empty, pristine, looking kind of like a **white rabbit in a snowstorm.** Kind of terrifying, really, if you think about it — like Kurt Vonnegut's character Billy Pilgrim, unstuck in time. Remember how nature abhors a vacuum?

That's because a vacuum is not a comfortable place. But alas, it can be a pretty common one.

To avoid it, it might help to reflect on the advice of another of my interviewees, who said, "It's better to start thinking about it *well before* you retire. Think about the *change* that's coming. Start processing ahead of time."

That's partly where the exercise above comes in. You'll get to make use of your list, edit as needed, and move forward as the book progresses.

The immediate and indispensable antidote to this void is adding a modicum of *structure and scheduling* to your life. Get out that newly pristine calendar and put in some *regular* items like reading/listening to the news, doing the daily crossword, going to the gym, writing a blog, even taking out the garbage. The trick is to develop some kind of daily routine that includes *doing* but also *being* — the latter including things like meditating, feeling consciously grateful, or developing a spiritual life (more on that in chapter sixteen, Be Fully).

Some people will want more structure, others less. I need only a little bit myself. So I have my morning routine of breakfast, reading email, and a shower; dealing with dirty dishes in the kitchen sink at the end of the day; taking out the garbage/recycling on Thursday nights; trimming my beard and doing the laundry Saturday mornings; and paying the credit card bills (fully!) at the end of the month. Not very much, eh? But this is where I started before adding Tapas, which imposed their own structure. I quickly added a workout, which I decided to do twice a week at whatever time of day felt best. Then I realized that I could have one meal a day, most days, with my wife. In the morning, we agree on which one it will be. (If we don't do this, our days don't overlap.)

Structure can come in many forms. Some people like creating lists and better organizing their world. Pick what works for *you*. The point is that imposing some structure is quite helpful to avoid a feeling of being untethered. And believe me, you don't want to get to the untethered place. So start filling in that snow-white calendar.

But be sure to leave some snow-white space since it's great to finally have the time to jump into something as it strikes you, to have flexibility, to have room to explore, for the unknown, the emergent. It may take awhile before you become accustomed to the possibility of doing something spur-of-the-moment, yet as long as your calendar has white space, this wonderful option will be open to you. I remember a summer day a couple of years ago when I noticed that the weather was great in San

Francisco — unusual for that time of year. Coincidentally, I also had an open calendar until late afternoon. I chose to do something I'd always wanted to: I rode my bike the 35 miles to the Ferry Building on the waterfront, had lunch, and then took the train (bike and all) home. Awesome day — and totally unplanned!

In the same vein, my friend Marc talked about how he keeps Friday open as an "anything day." And he has some structure, too: He devotes weekends to helping his wife with whatever tasks she has for him and does structured exercise with a trainer on Tuesdays and Thursdays. Garbage out Monday. Walk to dog park twice a week. Useful structure.

Another example of the balance between emergent and structured is Charlie, a longtime finance guy, who said he has some very full days and some wide-open days — and that he averages about three activities a day (I love that a longtime finance guy has computed this!). Every afternoon at 4:00, he does an hour and a half of cardio or weights, which has him feeling and looking good. He naps several afternoons a week (which research has recently shown is good for heart health). Much of the rest of his calendar is emergent.

Jim and his wife have designated Tuesday as "Date Day" and make no plans for that day without agreement. And he has other structured activities in his weeks, including morning news and email. That said, most of their time is "ad hoc punctuated by trying to find a day to do something spontaneously." Even folks who create a life without much structure at all need *some* structure. Moving to a shared calendar in the cloud simplified this couple's scheduling.

Be creative! Tom and Kathy drink alcohol only in the Friday-evening-to-Sunday-evening window to "avoid the weight and ending up as sots." And they read the Sunday paper in bed together over a bottle of champagne — every week! They do the crossword and Jumble together every day. Tom attends regular meetings of a men's group. Of course, time is also left open and unstructured, resulting in such delights as a spur-of-the-moment wading tour of the Everglades (hopefully sans crocagators!).

By and by, more structure will evolve. For years, I drove 50 miles every Monday, then back home, for a business meeting with the team at a start-up where I served as part-time CEO. For years, I served on the board and exec committee for a large synagogue and had monthly meetings for both. I now have periodic calls with my Leadership group and with a financial firm whose board I'm on.

There are also quarterly meetings for a nonprofit's board. And I practice piano for about an hour and a half pretty much every day (though not in any set time slot — for me, *some* structure is good, *more* structure is not), plus I go to a piano lesson every Tuesday. In any given week I'll have a couple or three appointments to do Life Coaching or Executive Coaching, so those also occupy a variable space on my calendar. And I lay in a lunch or two with a friend every week to stay in touch. Don't want to forget about some social activity with my wife and family or friends.

Speaking of social activity, one of the people I spoke with, Marte, worked and traveled a lot as a consultant during her Long Career. She has always been social, and now, she has a scheduled Friday activity: an open house for friends, so she can enjoy their company (more in chapter seven, Social Connection). She's even continued this via Zoom during Covid-19.

Inspect yourself for how much structure *you* need and put it in place ASAP — don't let the white rabbit get you, and don't put in more than you actually want. As long as you don't overcommit, you can tweak as you go. And if you *do* get overcommitted, let folks know you're new at this new life and then, to twist the meme, just *undo* it.

Still in his Long Career, Ralph says, "We will have a not-fixed schedule. We'll be our own boss." I imagine that will feel mighty good. But I also hope he and his wife add some structure of their own making!

Exercise: What structure items will you put on your calendar? Where will they go? Will they be at set times or flexible? How much white space do you want to protect? This will help you defeat the white rabbit.

• • •

CHAPTER THREE

DO SOMETHING YOU LOVE!

Go out into the world with your passion and
love for what you do, and just never give up.

— Dianne Reeves,
American jazz singer

With the sine qua non of structure taken care
of, it's time to let yourself out of the box
and **enjoy not having a full-time job.** It
shocks me how many conversations I've had with people
who have worked so hard for so long that they say they
have no idea what they'd love to do. But there must be
something. One person said, "This is relief from the stress
of work, an opportunity to be freer, to explore."

My COO and Group VP from years ago, who was a Marine drill sergeant back in the day, took up painting lessons after he left the electronics industry. Who would've guessed?

Maybe exploring leads you to a hobby you gave up years ago, or one you've always wanted to get into. Or something else you've longingly thought about from your past, like a sport you're excited to get back in shape for. It doesn't have to lead to the Olympics!

A fellow named Tim loved long-distance running, but didn't have the time. After his Long Career, he began doing 10Ks and then half-marathons and then marathons, including the Boston Marathon. This also helped sustain his health, and he continues to live fully decades later, even keeping up with his grandkids rather well.

Or maybe you're excited about getting into bridge or poker or mahjong.

Or taking up cooking or craft beer (drinking or making) or an artistic endeavor.

Marte finally had time to be the equestrienne she had always wanted to be. She cares for her horse, rides, and loves everything about the milieu. Plus, she has had more time to spend with her dogs, which delights her.

Could be writing — a blog, a book, an article — is calling your name. Or a role or two in community theater. Or teaching or giving talks about something you know a lot about.

David, a retired lawyer, took up native plant gardening and now has one of the most extensive native plant gardens in his area — practically a full-blown botanical garden.

Several people I interviewed also talked about this being a good time for doing some genealogy work, building family trees and such. This is perhaps part of reflecting on the fact that one day we, too, will become ancestors.…

What's important is to pick something you believe you'll enjoy. If you find you don't after all, pick something different. Eventually, you'll happen upon something that's a pleasure, that feels gratifying or fulfilling, or in some other way makes you smile.

Consider:

- ✓ How do you like to spend your free time?
- ✓ What kind of charitable organizations do you like to support?

✓ What is it you like about the places you visit?

✓ What have you daydreamed about doing if you had a bunch of free time and/or money?

✓ What do you like to learn about (via reading or TV or movies or podcasts, or the web, or whatever)? Learning and growing are hugely energizing!

✓ What do you know a lot about that you'd like to share with others (via writing/blogging, giving talks, podcasts, videos, or however)?

✓ What do you do for others that makes you feel good about yourself?

✓ What might you do with your spouse or your kid or a friend or a group of friends, whether travel, play cards/games, do sports, listen to or play music, hike, walk, jog, bike, or cook?

✓ Anything else that comes to mind!

In my case, it took 18 months (perhaps I was a little burned out?) after I became housedad before I woke up with the energy to start into something new: piano. I'd dabbled since my teens, but it had always felt slow and difficult. Now, finally, piano lessons beckoned me. My teacher has a bunch of kid students (she had been our kids' teacher!) and about a dozen adults. We grown-ups play a recital for each other at the teacher's house a few times a year, and for the first few years, my hands shook almost uncontrollably. After all those years of being good at what I did, I was suddenly a tyro, a mere newbie. It's now 16 years later and I'm not so bad at the ivories; it has been quite a journey and most assuredly a splendid one that wouldn't have *fit* during my Long Career.

ML has another artistic love: working on films, editing, and collaborating with others. He's now a partner in a video production company (see chapter eight on Keeping Your Business Brain Alive) and enjoys the energy of working with his 20-something partners. He also hangs out with people in the video world, which is great for social connection (see chapter seven on Social Connection).

The point is to find something you love and give it a shot. You don't have to be great at it; you just have to want to try. Enjoy it for what it does for you. Explore parts of you that have been dormant or barely present. Or give something completely new and different a chance; maybe it'll grab you. **In a recurring theme we'll see** (in chapter fifteen, Fail Freely, and elsewhere)**, for the first time in your life, there's no pressure to "succeed."** That's the beauty of it!

Exercise: What are two things you *really love* doing (review any list you may have built so far)? What is it you love about each of them? What do you feel when you're doing each of them? What are three ways you can get rolling on each of them (the three ways can be different for each activity). Start in on one, or, if you haven't yet finished your Long Career, jot these juicy action items down so they'll be ready for you when you're free.

• • •

CHAPTER FOUR

PLAYING CATCH-UP

Out of clutter, find simplicity.

— Albert Einstein,
Genius

Life can be pretty hectic during the Long Career phase. Afterward, though, there's time available. As noted, first put in some structure (you don't want to become untethered!), then start doing something you love (it's a reward — you deserve it!). Next, it's time to **catch up on all the stuff that has needed your attention for years.**

The most important thing on the list is to be sure your will or trust documents are current — or to actually draw some up if you haven't done so. Turns out none of us are immortal. Your family will be so much better off if you have these documents in place and up to date. If you don't act on this and somehow die, your loved ones will have to go through all sorts of machinations to pick up the financial pieces — awful for them to experience both the loss of you *and* these problems. Don't dally.

If you have plenty of assets, consider putting them into a trust, with the appropriate documents, and the necessary change-of-ownership documentation. Find a lawyer, pay them a few grand, and take care of your family prospectively. If you have a trust you created years ago, update it — laws have changed, and you may no longer want the same executor/executrix and/or successor trustee(s). If you had a sprinkling trust, if your kids are now responsible grown-ups, you may not want that anymore. Remember: These are not "file and forget" documents — they need to be kept current.

If you have IRA accounts (regular or Roth), make sure they have beneficiaries listed! Make sure you or your attorney or someone else will make clear to your beneficiaries what their options are for receiving these funds after you're gone. If you have life insurance or a pension plan, make sure beneficiaries are up to date there, too.

If you have only modest assets, be sure you at least have a will, so your assets go to the person you choose and relatives don't end up fighting over who gets what.

Equally important is a durable power of attorney for health care. This is the key document that catalogs what you'd like to happen if you experience nasty health outcomes that fall short of killing you. The more specific you can be about different sorts of possibilities, and what you'd want to happen in those instances, the better. The less you describe, the more you leave your loved ones to "deal with it." Not a great gift for them to receive while you are deeply in the tank. Note that some states have a standardized form you can use (in California, it's a booklet), and you may even be required to use the form rather than draw up a separate legal document. These can be free or very inexpensive, so everyone who cares about not leaving awful decisions to their spouse and/or kids at the worst possible time should have one!

The above is the "first things first" part of catching up. Next comes catching up on finances.

If you haven't done your post–Long Career financial planning, get it done! This is true whether you're a person of great or modest means. There are countless books on money and retirement — this is not one of them. I'm actually pretty good at this area, so I will nevertheless suggest the very least thing you need to do for yourself: Create a spreadsheet (computer or paper) with two columns. One column has your expectations of post–Long Career income. This can be money coming in from Social Security or other pensions, from investments, from work you do for pay (consulting, projects, coaching, part-time work, etc.), and any Required Minimum Distributions (RMDs) from IRAs, 401(k)s, and other such instruments. If you have after-tax savings/investments of other varieties that you plan to draw down over some period of years, count those, too. Taken together, that's what you'll have coming in.

Ralph says he'll "work long enough to ensure that the money doesn't run out." Good financial planning is the only path to understanding what that looks like.

Jim has taken this to the limit, having worked out a cash-flow plan that goes through his 100th birthday. He and his wife do monthly budget reviews to make sure things stay on track and that bad outcomes are avoided.

One piece of advice: Be conservative! That way, in good years, you'll have extra income you can enjoy, and in bad years, you'll still be OK. And keep in mind that "bad years" may very well appear unexpectedly, owing to unpredictable medical costs, so be sure to have a goodly fund to cover these. Or live it up, knowing full well that later you'll be paying the piper with hard times and financial challenges. It's a choice — one that's yours to make.

Geni said her partner's breast cancer and her own back surgery were unexpected expenses. And the bad economy from 2008 to 2010 was likewise not good news. That led to unanticipated and unwelcome cutbacks in their expenses. These things do happen, so make sure you've got some slack in your plan.

In the other column, list all your expenses, including income taxes you'll be paying. That includes mortgage/rent, medical, food, vacations, entertainment, home maintenance, car-related expenses, utilities, communications, insurance of all forms, real estate and car taxes, charitable giving, and anything else that applies to you.

The Income column must be greater than or equal to the Expenses column. If it isn't, you need to reduce items in the Expenses column (but not income taxes you'll owe — you'll be paying those regardless) until your budget is balanced. If you do this, you'll be in good shape. If you don't do this, you'll have bad surprises that can make an otherwise very rich and rewarding phase of life feel stressful and problematic.

Tom said the financial meltdown of 2009 was certainly stressful, "but we weathered it." If you plan for such things, you will, too.

As Joel, a fellow I interviewed, noted: "Withdrawal from cash flow had to be learned."

If you're not good at this type of analysis, pay someone to do it for you. But don't pay someone who will then recommend investments to you, because they won't give you an impartial analysis (especially now that the law has been changed so they no longer have a duty to advise you in a way that serves *your* best interests). More often than not, they'll push you in a direction that's in *their* best interest.

As I noted, I am decent at these financial matters, but I still went and found a financial advisor who charged a flat fee of a few hundred bucks an hour to analyze my analysis of our finances, just to make sure I wasn't missing something important. She did a great job, pointed out a few things to think about or dig into further, and left me with more peace of mind. It might be difficult to find a financial advisor who works strictly on a per-hour basis and who therefore doesn't push investments at you, but it's certainly worth the hunt.

Oh, and you'll want to contemplate when to start receiving Social Security retirement payments. Since these increase 8 percent per year each year you wait past your "full retirement age," it's likely best to wait until you're 70. To me, the best plan (if you've saved well in 401(k) accounts and IRAs and such) is to wait until the year after you turn 70.5 (or even 72 under recent tax law changes) to start your retirement account Required Minimum Distributions and planned investment drawdowns, then add them to your Social Security retirement benefits to make up your "nut" — the amount that, before taxes, yields enough after-tax dollars to cover all your planned expenses. This is a nice deal if you can get there. If not, be careful not to use up your retirement monies too soon (the "standard" advice given by books and articles I've read is to use a maximum of 4 percent of your retirement assets per year), and be careful not to let expenses get out of hand.

By the way, if, for your family's security, you've been carrying term life insurance for, say, the past 20 years, and its expiration is on the horizon, you'll find out that to renew, premiums will jump dramatically (six times higher in my case!). Unless you have some compelling reason otherwise, it's likely best to just let these policies go at this point.

One last thing to consider financially: long-term care insurance. This insurance pays when you're not able to do several of the so-called Activities of Daily Living (ADL), like getting dressed, eating, etc. It can pay a per-diem maximum toward care expenses for a set number of years or until death, and it may have benefits that escalate in line with inflation or not. This insurance is almost reasonable if one starts in one's 50s, and predictably gets progressively more expensive the later one starts. Also, the companies that offer the insurance have found that they have significantly underestimated what they have to pay out. So our premiums have gone up 30 percent and then subsequently doubled from there over the past few years (yeah, they say they'll "try" not to raise premiums…) L. But if one contemplates the nightmare of watching life savings evaporate while paying for the care of a largely incapacitated loved one for years and years, one might consider long-term care insurance to be a very prudent investment.

In an alternative approach to these risks, ML put some annuities in place in case Alzheimer's set in, since there's some on both sides of his family. He now feels that their needs for the future are "well accounted for and that this helps with emotional stability."

A further forward-looking move at this point if you have grandkids and the means is to consider gifting some funds into a 529 plan to grow tax-free for educational expenses; if you start when they're smallish, they'll be in great shape later.

Please remember that I'm not a financial advisor or a tax guy, so do your homework with your accountant and/or financial advisor and/or estate planner and/or tax guy.

A woman I spoke with, Jane, hired a financial consultant three years before she anticipated wrapping up her Long Career. She put appropriate plans in place (and, yes, drew up a trust document and durable power of attorney for health care) and then felt secure about the future. Guess what? Five years later, she still feels that way!

And then, of course, there are other items that will need attention, now that you've finally got the time. You needn't address everything right away, but instead, try to nibble away at them. For example, we remodeled portions of our house in three phases, and then added a fourth phase for landscaping, over a period of two-and-a-half years — a leisurely pace.

Your home may also need all manner of repairs, from paint to a new roof. It's typical that this sort of deferred maintenance is exactly that: deferred. Now there's finally time to fix the things that very much need fixing, or to pursue any dreams you've had about what you'd like to do to create your dream home — add a room, move a wall, put in a sauna. You could choose to spruce the place up, transform a grown kid's room into a studio, and generally make your place more for adults only. You could turn a former home office into a guest room so when friends (or grown kids) visit, they'll feel welcome and pampered — like adults, even! Maybe another room turns into a quiet reading space. (Full disclosure: Our house used to have two bedrooms for our kids; now we have a guest room *and* an office.)

A fellow I know named Craig really, really enjoys doing projects around the house. He has a long list accumulated and is looking forward to getting to it once he has finished his Long Career.

It's easy to imagine that bathrooms and the kitchen could use updating, appliances replacing, and so on. If you've got the funds and the inclination, take these tasks on. Please know that they can even be fun since you're not trying to jam the work into the middle of your Long Career and parenting responsibilities. These home-improvement activities work especially well if you don't impose some artificial deadline like "it'll be done by Thanksgiving," which can make the effort stressful and challenging. Anyone who's ever done one of these projects knows they never end "on time." Better to approach them as "who cares when they're complete" as long as, say, the house isn't a disaster area for longer than is tolerable. If you can limit the work to certain areas at a time, then time can be flexible.

Jim and his wife (who married after becoming widower and widow) remodeled their home extensively to make it more suitable to their combined adult needs, and to provide separate living space for a grown child.

Then there's landscaping, replacing a deck or a walkway, adding outdoor lighting. Now you have the time available to pursue these possibilities, either through your own handy actions or by wielding your credit card.

Moving beyond the above, there's also *your* stuff. If you're one of the few with a well-organized garage that's used for your car(s), good on you. If you're not, now's the time to give things away to others who need and can benefit from them. In fact, the same is true for objects throughout your house. Cleaning out clutter and giving stuff away may well leave you feeling emotionally lighter, too. Donate old clothes, thin out knick-knacks, release all manner of stuff you haven't used in years. When my dad died, he still had a dozen unopened boxes of notes from college and grad school — not needed anymore! This effort has a further benefit: The more you get rid of, the less your family will have to deal with if you eventually have to move to assisted living or when you die.

Marte pointed out that she "just doesn't need *things* so much anymore" and so has done "lots of decluttering."

My piano teacher says she wants to rid her garage of accumulated stuff to help her kids avoid the cleanup burden one day.

Kathy and Tom departed to warmer climes after their Long Careers, so they "cleared out a lot of old stuff in order to start fresh."

I really recommend you do the first-things-first and financial aspects of catch-up without fail and without delay. Other items will likely be rewarding and can certainly be done at one's chosen pace, however leisurely.

Amusingly, one person I interviewed said that "anticipation of catching up on these tasks was more rewarding than the doing." Others admitted that they have so much going on after their Long Careers that they *still* haven't started doing their catch-up items — like Geni, who completed her Long Career 15 years ago, but confessed that what she had caught up on was "not so much!"

Let me say it again because it's *soooo* important: Do the first-things-first and financial aspects of catch-up without fail and without delay. This is the only place in the book I repeat myself.

CHAPTER FIVE

ADD TAPAS AND STIR

Eighty percent of success is showing up.

— Woody Allen,
American director,
writer, and actor

I miss 100 percent of the shots I never take.

— Wayne Gretzky,
Canadian hockey
player and coach

Ninety percent of the game is mental.
The other half is physical.

— Yogi Berra,
American baseball
player

You've added structure, treated yourself to starting in on something you love, embarked on some catch-up work, and now, if you feel like it, **you can start adding Tapas to your life.**

A few years ago, I was co-leading a seminar called "How to Get the Life You Want." During one of the exercises, we went around to each of the 15 to 20 people in the room, asking, "What's next for *you?*" A very poignant moment came when two people sitting next to each other, a 60-something just-retired high school teacher and a 20-something just-graduating college student, offered virtually the same answer: "Gee, I don't really have much of a clue." Turns out that these two times of life are not dissimilar.

Of course, the new "retiree" has an advantage: They don't have to figure out how to get a job, build a family, pay the rent/mortgage, and prove their utility to society; plus, they have a lifetime of experience to draw on.

Which means there's very little risk to **just adding a Tapa,** and then seeing whether it satisfies you and keeps you craving more. If you like it, let it nourish you until you're satiated (if you ever are), at which time you can move on to the next. The very nice context is that this phase isn't your Long Career; very little is riding on it.

You can just try things and see what happens. So step out and be adventurous — there's nothing to lose but a little time, which you've now got in abundance. Worse comes to worst, you'll have learned what may inform future Tapa selections. Learning stretches you and, viewed propitiously, is just plain fun!

If that's not how you roll, I suggest trying **a tool that will help you assess whether or not a Tapa might be to your liking.** Take yourself to https://www.viacharacter.org/survey/account/register and click on Take the Free VIA Survey. (You'll have to register, but I've never had any subsequent contact from them, though they may of course change those policies at any time.) Your results will be what *they* call your Character Strengths, rank-ordered from most to least salient. *I* think of these as the things that *give you juice*. When you're using those, life tends to be good. When you aren't, not so much.

I've included the top four items on my own VIA survey results, below. If you already have a few (or many) Tapas that you're considering adding to your life, you can use *your* top VIA results as a litmus test to see how the different possibilities might work out for you. As an example, let's walk through how *my* top VIA items help me select Tapas.

VIA Survey of Character Strengths

Here are your scores on the VIA Survey of Character Strengths. For how to interpret and use your scores, see the book Authentic Happiness. The ranking of the strengths reflects your overall ratings of yourself on the 24 strengths in the survey, how much of each strength you possess. Your top five, especially those marked as Signature Strengths, are the ones to pay attention to and find ways to use more often.

Your Top Strength

Gratitude
You are aware of the good things that happen to you, and you never take them for granted. Your friends and family members know that you are a grateful person because you always take the time to express your thanks.

Your Second Strength

Appreciation of beauty and excellence
You notice and appreciate beauty, excellence, and/or skilled performance in all domains of life, from nature to art to mathematics to science to everyday experience.

Your Third Strength

Curiosity and interest in the world
You are curious about everything. You are always asking questions, and you find all subjects and topics fascinating. You like exploration and discovery.

Your Fourth Strength

Humor and playfulness
You like to laugh and tease. Bringing smiles to other people is important to you. You try to see the light side of all situations.

Gratitude: If a Tapa gives me the opportunity to thank people, provides me the chance to be grateful and thankful, I feel good. Clearly, almost any possibility would yield some of this, but others might well have more. I apply Gratitude in all my Tapas.

Appreciation of Beauty and Excellence: I'm very visual, and when what I see is pleasing, that delights me, whether art, nature, people, or objects. I also take pleasure in seeing others at the top of their capabilities. So going to a fabulous piano concert feels terrific. In contrast, a Tapa where ugliness is all around and people aren't bringing their A-game (following crass politicians on Twitter — ugh) is definitely not for me. I apply this "strength" to everything around me all the time. Some might say that when I'm doing that, I'm being *mindful* — more on that later.

Curiosity and Interest in the World: I'm like a 10-year-old inside, always curious, always seeking to learn something. If a Tapa is plain and simple and entirely known to me, there's not much joy in that. If there's newness for me, and it's an interesting variety of newness, that works well. I apply this tenet to all my Tapas, as there's so much to learn wherever one looks. One example is my Coaching Tapa, which gives me a deep window into another person, with the added variety that comes from dealing with different individuals —notwithstanding that our work is for *their* benefit. Another example is my Reading/Learning Tapa. I read the ScienceDaily.com website every day and subscribe to *Science News* (a fine, short magazine). Both help me keep up with what's going on in my areas of interest (yes, it's work to get beyond the sensational news headlines about the worst 1 percent of everything). I also make sure I periodically head off on tangents. At the moment, I'm diving into the Google Arts & Culture Grand Tour of Italy, and immersed in a long Wikipedia article on Christianity (started because I wondered about the differences between different strands of Christianity).

Humor and Playfulness: For better or for worse, my brain is always coming up with mischief and silliness (and puns). Most of them, thankfully for those around me, are left in my braincase. But I do let some out, and I try to include people in my life who appreciate them, or who at least like to play around a little. If a potential Tapa is full of stiff, humorless folks, that won't work for me. In my *Travel* Tapa, for instance, when my wife and I were in Ireland, we discovered that seemingly *everyone* there was willing to joke around, have a laugh, be playful. Awesome place. (Plus, there was good gluten-free beer everywhere. Since I developed an allergy to gluten at 48 after a horrible virus, maybe I should move to Ireland? It was challenging to live gluten-free 20 years ago since there were few products available and eateries didn't really know about it at the time. Nowadays it seems pretty easy.)

Geni also places high value on "curiosity and interest in the world" and has assembled a variety of Tapas, including some consulting, work on a local Board, some medical forensics work, two writing courses, travel with friends, being an audience for her partner's equestrian activities, and singing. "Gotta keep learning!" she told me.

Another way to home in on potentially satisfying Tapas is to discover whether you're a convergent or divergent thinker.

Convergent thinkers tend to like to gather whatever data they feel is absolutely needed, and then make a decision. They like things to be settled and clear. For these folks, it can be downright difficult to let an issue continue to be "open" without deciding on it ASAP. Making a decision is what's satisfying. In contrast, divergent thinkers gather some data, which leads to more data to be gathered, and then yet more; the decision is often put off as long as possible, sometimes past the deadline of interest. For them, making a decision can be agony, since there is always more information to be gathered that *could possibly* be useful. These are both fine flavors of human, and we definitely benefit from both!

As with all things, though, there's a continuum. But whatever you are — Divergent or Convergent or anything in between — it's a good trait to keep in mind as you choose your Tapas (never mind your Long Career). For instance, you wouldn't want to be in the pit of a stock exchange making hundreds of split-second decisions a day if you are a divergent thinker. And being a researcher may not be a great fit for a strong convergent thinker.

When it comes to the transition to a Tapas Life, divergent thinkers might find the process very natural. They roll along, opportunities appear, and they grab those that suit them when they suit them. They're OK with letting their life be very emergent, for things to arise organically. In contrast to one's Long Career, which often demands that decisions be made, the Tapas Life may feel liberating to a

Divergent. Of course, as in all Tapas Life recipes, you can add as much or as little structure as you wish, so not everything need be wide open. That said, I've met Divergents who find it difficult to just fall into a new Tapa, instead feeling somewhat immobilized by the degree of freedom now available to them. The solution to this, I believe, is adopting what's called a *rapid-prototyping* mentality: Try something. If you like it, keep it; otherwise, let it go and try something else. Reminding yourself that there's no significant risk or downside may make it easier to just jump in. **Any action at all on any Tapa will prove better and more useful than remaining frozen in indecision.**

If you're a Convergent, you might find the transition to a Tapas Life to be more of a challenge. In your Long Career, you might've found the structure the world provides to be a comfortable thing. You're perhaps used to goals and deadlines and making decisions about how to achieve them. Most important, how you spend the bulk of your waking hours is something that has been settled for decades through the rigors of your Long Career as well as time with family. You may find the sudden arrival of the blank calendar to be very daunting indeed.

I noted the example of the medical doctor in chapter two, White Rabbit in a Snowstorm. Most doctors have had a huge portion of their time scheduled over the past

30+ years. All that time, they've also been making decisions. Their Long Career's attributes have prescribed (sorry, non-punners) what their days have looked like. Then comes the next phase: terra incognita, where nothing is settled. Of course, by and by, they can get on with gathering data and making decisions about what they want their lives to look like and wind up feeling very fulfilled and satisfied. I'm merely noting the challenging nature of their transition — it's a pretty major change!

Other Convergents may or may not have a similarly disorienting transition ahead of them, but they are likely to experience the arrival of a blank calendar as more of a hurdle than a Divergent.

One other heads-up to Convergents: You might experience life after your Long Career to be a lot less efficient, which can take some time to get comfortable with. But if you *can* get comfortable with it, you may well find it pretty tasty to be able to enjoy the slack times and opportunities for spontaneity and observation/contemplation.

Lastly, Convergents may also find themselves feeling frozen in front of a choice, though for them that may well be from its not being obvious what the minimum necessary data to make a decision *is*. Just as with the Divergents, taking **any action at all on any Tapa will prove more useful than remaining frozen in place.**

One surefire way to find the right Tapas Life for you: Think about the things you already know a lot about or have a lot of experience with or wish you did. Look for ways to get involved in those. Join a related group. Do some consulting or project work. Write/blog/podcast about it. Get friends together to do it. Give a talk on it. Teach it. Take a course in it to go even deeper. Start a business around it. Most important: **Try to avoid thinking about everything that could "not work" about it and just get started,** for goodness' sake!

Because if you don't try, you won't find out what could possibly turn out to be wonderful.

If it doesn't turn out to be wonderful, mine the experience for learning, which will help you with your next pick. This is a time of life when having something not work out can be just fine (see chapter fifteen, Fail Freely).

Marc is a good example of someone who modeled his Tapas out of his Long Career expertise. As an architect (for part of his career), he often had ideas for making sculptures, but no time to actually create them. Now he does, and he's expanded his repertoire to include painting, origami, paper-cutting, and more. "I'm happy — but didn't intentionally assemble this life. I just took one thing from here and one thing from there. It's just cobbled together. I like the idea of the Tapas Life."

If you find yourself unable to start in on *any* Tapa, you may have some mental script or belief you are subconsciously using to hold yourself back. Perhaps you think you don't deserve this much freedom, or that trying something new is far too risky, or that you don't really know what you want. It's amazing how many limiting mental models/assumptions/beliefs there can be. To get yourself over this hurdle, try working through this with people close to you. And know that you truly can do this.

MJ Elmore has four broad Tapas: oil painting (her *flow* activity — see chapter sixteen on Being Fully); philanthropy that is particularly focused on a variety of people who will greatly benefit; investing (see chapter eight on Keeping Your Business Brain Alive); and working to motivate women. As full as her life is now, she notes that it was tough to "get off the bus" of her attractive career in venture capital. Attending Stanford University's Distinguished Careers Institute (DCI) served as a springboard for launching her post–Long Career life; it aims to help renew purpose, build community, and recalibrate wellness for people who have concluded their Long

Career. Incidentally, the program also gained her a network of interested and interesting peers.

Once you've added one Tapa to your life, when the muse strikes you, add another. And continue until you're starting to feel busier than you wish. That's when you may want to discard a Tapa, add a different one, or leave more open time on your calendar for whatever grabs you in the moment.

Some Tapas last for years or even forever. Some are temporary and time-bound (I did menial tasks and walked neighborhoods for a Congressional campaign for six months; this did *not* feed my VIA Survey items, but it very much needed doing). Others may appeal for a while and then lose their luster. There's a great deal of flexibility in how you assemble your Tapas collection over time. Learning, nourishing your personal growth, and feeding your life energy feels good at any age.

Doug said that when he was 50, he would've guessed he'd be retired and playing golf. At 70, he says, "Some days I think I'll have to go back to work to get some free time!" His Tapas have included writing a book, running for and being elected to his local school board (and then becoming its president), raising money for a clinic for his town, and then joining the clinic's board. He has an

Exercise Tapa (biking), and at the time I spoke with him, he was looking to join a local chorus. Divorced, he was also lucky to reconnect with a high school sweetheart (who "married — and divorced! — the other guy"), and now he has a new family. His philosophy is to "network and open yourself up to possibility."

Multiple people I spoke with observed that while there's a lot more time available post–Long Career, it can sometimes seem as if there's actually *less* — because it just flies by (that's where mindfulness comes in; more on this in chapter sixteen on Being Fully)! Often, folks tell me they don't understand how they ever managed to have time in their days for their Long Career.…

Suzanne likes hiking and biking and has a long list of books to read. She'd like to put herself in a big city for a week every month — just to enjoy the energy, the vibe, all that's available there. But, like MJ, above, she's finding that while she'd like to "put the brakes on, the money's easy now," so she's having to make a real effort to taper business in favor of some tasty Tapas.

Craig loves restoring old cars. He's got two teed up: One needs its engine rebuilt, and the other, in his words, needs *everything*. A terrific Tapa for him that will last many years.

As Ralph nears retirement, he says that he's usually taken life as it comes, and views retirement as "just a life phase." He imagines golf, tennis, skiing. Traveling sounds good, but he "gets antsy" if he's away from home more than two weeks. More time with family. Maybe some volunteer work. He expects to do more of what he *wants* to do versus things he *has* to do. "It will be nice to get up and say, 'I can decide what I want to do today.'" He also wants to cook more, and do so "with pizzazz!" This is an early view of a whole collection of Tapas just waiting for Ralph to sample.

Please hear again that it doesn't matter if you "fail" miserably at a Tapa you try. This may well be the first time in your life that if something turns out poorly, there are no big stakes, no nasty consequences. Instead, there's simply the opportunity to learn something from the experience.

CHAPTER SIX

• • •

REVIEW

A good goal is like a strenuous
exercise — it makes you stretch.

— Mary Kay Ash, founder/CEO,
Mary Kay Cosmetics

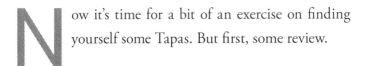ow it's time for a bit of an exercise on finding
yourself some Tapas. But first, some review.

- What structure have you installed in your life
  to avoid feeling untethered? Do you need to add
  more? What might that be? Conversely, if your
  life feels too structured, what might you remove?
- What in your life needs catching up on? Updating
  legal documents or a financial spreadsheet?

Renewing relationships with family and friends? Long-postponed home repairs? Consider making a short list of items to catch up on, and then tackle the top two. Be assured — it will feel terrific to finally cross them off your list.

- Have you started doing something you love? Time's a-wastin'! Carve out a couple of hours and have at it. Doesn't matter if you're good at it or bad at it. Doesn't matter what others think (although they're most likely to be envious that you're getting to do it). Doesn't even matter if you find out you don't love it after all; in that case, learn from the trial and move on to something else. You'll for sure find something you love after enough attempts, and it will have been worth the journey.

- Once you've taken the VIA Survey, list half a dozen Tapas you might want to try. Now take them one at a time and see how they feed or don't feed your top four or five VIA Survey priorities. What you discover may strengthen your interest in adding a Tapa or two and make you think twice about some of the others. If the items on your list don't seem to do much toward feeding your VIA Survey priorities, you'll probably want to reflect on whether your list contains items you think you *should* pursue, rather than ones that would truly feed you. This brings to mind a Chinese proverb often quoted by my friend Sandra: "Tension is who you think you should be. Relaxation is who you are."

• Build your list of potential Tapas from within and without — from conversations with and questions asked of others you respect. And get at it! Your very own bespoke Tapas Life may come together quickly or take several years to assemble (as mine did — but I didn't have the benefit of this book!) or something in between. But the path always starts with launching in on a Tapa and finding out if it's a keeper or merely a learning experience.

• • •

CHAPTER SEVEN

SOCIAL CONNECTION

Social connection is such a basic
feature of human experience that when
we are deprived of it, we suffer.

— Leonard Mlodinow,
*American theoretical
physicist, screenwriter,
and author*

ots of research has pointed to the perhaps obvious fact that we need connection with other humans to live a healthy life.

In fact, **your social connections (or lack thereof) can have the biggest impact on whether your post–Long Career life becomes an undesirable decline to death or whether you continue to live well.**

Several people I interviewed mentioned how much of their social connection came from the people they worked with. But they found that these relationships tapered off after their Long Career was over. They missed those connections, and that felt bad.

Imagine yourself fairly isolated. Sounds depressing, no? And that, in turn, has been shown to weaken one's immune system, resulting in increased mortality rates.

Social connection can come from family, friends, and acquaintances, and it needs to be pursued on a regular basis (i.e., getting together with other people on the holidays and your birthday is not sufficient). It doesn't happen by FM (f***ing magic) [thanks, Tracy G.]. You have to make an effort to reach out to people, and then you have to invest in the relationships.

Maybe if feels easiest to start fostering those connections with family — and not just with your immediate family, but also with relatives you didn't have the time to see over the years of your Long Career. There's that cousin you've always liked; now you could arrange to meet up. Or maybe there's a sibling you've always had a difficult relationship with; perhaps now is the time to work on it before one of you is dead.

I have an uncle I've always admired and enjoyed visiting. He was in the entertainment management business and always had a million stories. Yet when my dad died, I managed stupidly to piss this uncle off no end. And we didn't speak for 18 years. At the millennium, two years before ending my Long Career, I sent him a letter apologizing, saying I missed our relationship and that I hoped we could hit the reset button. He accepted. Somehow, until I could see the end of my Long Career on the near horizon, I embarrassingly didn't muster the energy it took to apologize. But it was so worth the effort when I finally took the initiative!

Then, of course, there are friends and acquaintances to cultivate, who can come in all sorts of flavors. Perhaps there are some people you like doing things with or spending time with in group situations, others you value for gabbing, and a few with whom you can go deep, whether discussing important issues of our times or baring your soul. If you're married, there are likely to be couple friends, if you're lucky; it's a great thing when two couples have the good fortune to truly click (each person really likes the three others), and it makes sense to be all in on those. By approaching these very special relationships with unconditional positive regard — always think the best of them, always give the benefit of the doubt, never be suspicious, always be there for them — all four of you will be handsomely rewarded.

My friend Jim and his wife have a monthly "Adventure Day" with another couple. Each month, it's one couple's turn to figure out an overnight within a three-hour drive at a set price limit. They pick up the other couple at noon, do the surprise/adventure overnight, and are home the next day by noon. Highly inventive social connection (try it!), plus it fulfills both Structure and Social Connection Tapas.

In the previous chapter, I talked about divergent and convergent thinkers. Another way one can categorize people is as primarily introverts or extroverts — and I am using these terms in a very particular way. Simply, an introvert is someone who *uses energy* to be with other people. An extrovert is someone who *gains energy* from being with other people. Both types can be gregarious, have apparently outgoing personalities, and seem rather social. But an introvert can only take so much stimulus; after being with others, they generally need to go someplace by themselves to recharge. Extroverts, by contrast, are generally happy to be with other people almost continuously (and being alone can suck the energy out of them). Whatever type sounds like you, however, rest assured that we all *need* social connection.

If you're an extrovert, it may feel easy to meet people — you pick up acquaintances everywhere. Introverts, by contrast, might need to expend more effort to make connections, but the effort is well spent. The most obvious way to increase the social bonds in your life is by joining a group, whether a spiritual community, a common-interest group (e.g., book club, foreign language group, movie-night group, wine-tasting club, a charitable organization like helping out at a food kitchen, a sports group like a swim or tennis club, or a softball league); or a civic group (like Rotary International). I've met several people who enjoy traveling with tour groups, where they've met interesting folks who have become their friends. These, of course, are just a few options, but being a joiner, even if it doesn't always feel natural, can lead to relationships that fill our essential human need for social connection.

You may well find that you have different sets of family and friends who you like to be with for different reasons, and it's a wonderful situation when you have cultivated a whole garden of friends (could be a handful of people or many) who together feed your assorted needs for social connection. I've even met some of my neighbors —don't forget your neighbors! — through an organized activity meant to help with emergency preparedness and environmental sustainability.

Whatever your source of connections, I can't stress enough how important this need is. **You simply *must* fulfill it to have a chance at a happy, healthy, long life.** Good article here, if you wish to learn more: http://sitn.hms.harvard.edu/flash/2018/loneliness-an-epidemic/

Technology can also lead to and cement social connections, as we all know from the Covid-19 pandemic. But ultimately, in-person, face-to-face connections are much more fulfilling. Even before the virus, my wife liked to enjoy a drink over FaceTime to keep up with a really good friend who lives halfway across the country.

Ultimately, whether you connect over the ether or in-person, what you get out of a relationship is a function of what you put into it. So be sure to put something — usually a mix of time, care, curiosity, and positive regard — into the ones you value.

• • •

CHAPTER EIGHT

KEEP YOUR BUSINESS BRAIN ALIVE

Experience is not what happens to you; it's
what you do with what happens to you.

— Aldous Huxley,
English writer and
philosopher

It is impossible to enjoy idling thoroughly
unless one has plenty of work to do.

— Jerome K. Jerome,
English writer

f your Long Career is ending soon or has already been
completed, you may well want to **think about how to**
leverage all the business-related knowledge you've
accumulated during those work years. This can serve

as good mental exercise, a path to social connection, and, possibly, a meaningful activity that benefits others. Not to mention you'll be reaping a dividend on your decades of work and learning.

You might do some consulting, special projects for people in your business area, advisory or board work, recruiting — the point is to keep using what you know, albeit in a more circumscribed, tapas-like fashion that leaves you time for discovery and enjoying more variety in your life.

Beyond keeping your days busy and interesting, if you have an ongoing need for additional income after your Long Career, there's nothing like small bites of paying work, and companies often need experienced consultants to take on projects, fill in for folks on parental leave, or simply provide otherwise absent expertise.

Geni noted that it's terrific to be able to pick and choose projects from those that come her way. And Marte also likes that she can be so selective — and earn a buck, to boot.

One caveat: These types of gigs can be less plentiful during a recession or slack times in the economy, unless it's a special "who you know" situation.

Your business brain may also prove useful in a mentoring role, which can be especially meaningful and gratifying. These can often be found in schools and colleges, or perhaps through former colleagues or work-related connections. I've occasionally offered and been called on by grown children of friends as a mentor, and it's been a real pleasure to get to know what's on the younger generation's mind and help out.

Marc talked about how he tutors young people on STEM subjects he used to teach — and especially appreciates the opportunity to be with people at an earlier stage than his own, which triggers all kinds of evocative memories for him.

After his huge Long Career job, a friend of mine in Texas now trains folks coming up the ranks, and is having a great time mentoring. Same for a local acquaintance who has moved from a real pressure-cooker job to advising, supporting, and developing others. In the process, these two are keeping their business brain alive and enjoying the gratifying work of bringing others along, too, while avoiding the jolt of going from decades of challenging work to zippo overnight. I've always thought it would be wonderful if more companies had the forethought to leverage the knowledge of their most experienced people to help grow others rather than pushing those super-capable people out the door, or waiting for them to exit totally spent.

You could also try on an entrepreneurial venture, although beware that these often wind up being all-consuming. But they can also be energizing and exciting, and there's always the possibility of taking them on for a while and then turning them over to a replacement you've hired for yourself, or selling the business, thereby recapturing your Tapas Life. Of course, in the process you may discover that you prefer having a second major career instead of a Tapas Life.

And then there's board and advisor work. Know that to do this for a business, you will very likely need to have been a high-level contributor and bring expertise and/or key contacts. To do this for a nonprofit, it's also typically expected that you will be a significant donor. These spots may appeal to you — or not.

One friend, Tom, tried doing some board work and also being president of his non-fancy golf club — and says "he won't do those again, either of them!" His Long Career, he adds, is "not missed at all, in any way, even an iota." And I say, Good for him.

I'll seize the moment here to again note that whatever your business-brain activity, if it "fails" or you hate it, that's OK — just learn from the experience and try something else (or even try the same thing again, now knowing what you know). The only exception is if you need a steady income, in which case you may need to make a *Business Tapa* — or several Business Tapas — work more predictably. If you have several sources of income, you can adventure a bit more and not care so much about outcomes.

• • •

CHAPTER NINE

MEANINGFUL WORK — GIVE SOMETHING BACK

Happiness comes when we test our skills
towards some meaningful purpose.

— John Stossel,
*American reporter
and libertarian pundit*

As far as we can discern, the sole purpose
of human existence is to kindle a light
in the darkness of mere being.

— Carl Jung,
*Swiss psychiatrist and
writer*

It is more blessed to give than to receive.

— Acts 20:35

From the time you were able to sit up, crawl, stand, feed yourself, use a toilet, and so on through all your education and well into your Long Career, you've had to prove your competence. You've had to show you can do it. As a kid, it's part of growing up. In the work world, it's necessary to secure advancement and more pay and perks (and power, if that's your thing).

Then, perhaps in your 40s or 50s, you might have looked in the mirror one morning and thought to yourself, "I'm competent — I no longer need to be constantly proving that!" (I have to add that the exception here may be if you're caught up in trying to prove yourself to a demanding parent, even one who has passed away. That's a topic for a different kind of book, and *Trapped in the Mirror: Adult Children of Narcissists in Their Struggle for Self,* by Elan Golomb, is a good one.)

Once you achieved that sense of competence in your work, it's possible you also felt your Long Career was slightly less interesting and fulfilling.

In his book *Transitions: Making Sense of Life's Changes,* William Bridges notes that **the first half of life is taken up with proving *competence*, and the second half with the search for *meaning.*** You may be ready to get started on that second half if you haven't already. Most activities that are meaningful tend to be about doing something selflessly for a person or a cause that directly or eventually benefits others. That's one reason many see parenting as the most meaningful thing they've ever done.

One person I interviewed told me that "satisfaction of others makes one happier than searching for satisfaction of my own." Another said, "I get more out of giving and helping others than out of anything else."

I'll admit that even after I'd put four years into assembling my own Tapas Life, and even though it was indeed excellent, there were times when it still felt *empty* at some level. This is when I learned about the need to find a *Meaningful* Tapa for myself — one outside my own family, since my kids were already off on their own by then and my wife is a powerhouse who is fully engaged in her work world. After aimlessly and fruitlessly bumbling around for perhaps six months, a lunch with an acquaintance who mentioned that he was thinking about becoming a life coach turned out to be the seed for my Meaningful Tapa. On my way home, I pondered the notion of his becoming a life coach; he was, I'll say, a *complicated* fellow. After a while, the thought popped into my head: "If he could be a life coach, *anybody* could be a life coach." And after a little more driving: "Heck, even *I* could be a life coach."

My wife suggested I read a book called *Coactive Coaching*, by Laura Whitworth, Karen Kimsey-House, Henry Kimsey-House, and Phillip Sandahl (I read the 2nd edition — it's now in its 4th, but I prefer the 2nd). As it turned out, I flew up to Lake Tahoe that weekend to visit with my brother, an avid skier. I don't ski much because I don't like the cold, and that weekend, it snowed seven feet — the perfect time for me to sit around the rental apartment reading the book, with pauses to gaze at the peaceful scene of beauty outside the window. I discovered that the life coaching concept fit me like a comfy old sweater. One thing I had enjoyed in my Long Career was developing people through coaching and mentoring. I liked engaging with another person on matters of depth and substance, and it seemed that life coaching work could refill that now-missing part of my life. So, soon after, I enrolled at the Coaches Training Institute (the founders wrote *Co-Active Coaching*), studied up, and got started. Nine years later, I'm still doing that (and some executive coaching as well). I find it very meaningful working with someone closely so they can learn more about themselves and move their life toward how they want it. Yet I still consider it a Tapa, not a new Long Career, so I cap my coaching at five active clients at any given moment, which leaves plenty of time and energy for my other Tapas, as well as anything new that might come along.

Of course, if you're searching for meaning, you can also choose to help a nonprofit organization you believe in, either as a volunteer or for pay. The more local the organization, the greater the chances you will get a close-up view of the good you're doing, thereby making it even more meaningful for you (and more likely that through it, you'll find more social connections — a twofer).

Suzanne volunteered for a local 4-H Club, working with multi-generational groups and disabled kids. As this activity involved horses, she found that she had reignited her childhood love of same. The kids win, and so does she.

Charlie the finance guy is chair of his church's investment committee. This is a triple-win: He's giving back while keeping his business brain alive and enjoying social connection. He also heads the capital campaign at a school.

I do have to add a word of caution about doing work for nonprofits. I discovered through hard-earned experience that they're not always run like businesses, where everyone knows they need to contribute to the growth and profitability of the company, and quickly, in order to progress in their careers. This can lead to what I've sometimes described as "jamming an hour's work into a month." If you're a decisive person of action, you may be surprised to find that things move along more slowly than you're used to. On the other hand, perhaps you're not from the dog-eat-dog business world, and your personal preference may be a fine fit for the nonprofit world. That said, there are definitely many excellent nonprofits that are run efficiently, effectively, and admirably well. So, just poke around and ensure you're choosing one that's right for you.

ML and his wife, JL, work on water-deficit issues up in Napa. "We don't want to leave the earth with problems," he says. And because the work is with neighbors, it also enriches their Social Connection Tapa.

Any challenges you encounter are well worth it, according to retired businesspeople I've spoken with who go the nonprofit or pro bono route. After his Long Career, David, an attorney who had already been doing a lot of good by resolving disputes for the state bar and running volunteer workshops, decided to give back after his retirement by litigating challenges to inadequate and/or unequal school system funding. Unsurprisingly, David said it felt great to work on behalf of kids' education — clearly very meaningful work.

Joel also decided to help children — in a big way. He raised $35 million and started a nondenominational college-prep high school to change kids' lives for the better. The endeavor took much of his active attention for 15 years — and he remains on the board to this day. This is both meaningful giving back and a *legacy* project.

Jim wound up with meaningful work he didn't seek out: caring for his wife as she battled cancer. Afterward, he did nonprofit work at a hospital, with a community foundation, and for the symphony.

Tom fell into one of his Tapas when he was asked to officiate at a friend's wedding. This was new territory for Tom, but he agreed, got ordained online (a curious aspect of the Internet Age), worked hard at putting together a ceremony that would delight the couple and be a good experience for guests, and was a big hit — so much so that other attendees asked Tom to do the same for them. They referred more friends, and today, his officiating skills — which he has developed into an art — are in great demand. He found a really *Meaningful* Tapa, loves the activity, gets a lot of social connection (see chapter seven), and makes good money. He does as much or as little of this work as he chooses, as he feels the urge.

Perhaps at the core of giving back is the feeling of being useful, of being needed, of having mattered — and

of doing something that matters. Ultimately, this Tapa really fills the post–Long Career raison d'être. So if you're going to have only a couple of Tapas, make sure one is *Meaningful*.

• • •

CHAPTER TEN

CHOOSE HEALTH

With age comes the understanding
and appreciation of your most
important asset: your health.

— Oprah Winfrey,
*American media
personality and
producer, actress,
and philanthropist*

S ince you're going to be around for another two
or three decades, consider paying great attention
to your health, to avoid experiencing the sort of
decline that can gradually curtail the scope of your life.

In addition to nurturing your social connections, this
means paying attention to eating and exercise.

I've always done OK at eating and exercise, but I became a lot more aware and focused after reading a book that's well worth your time: *Younger Next Year* by Chris Crowley and Henry S. Lodge, M.D. It's a fun read about a guy who is in lousy health and decides to do something about it. So he hunts for a partner in the effort and eventually finds his M.D. coauthor. And they ping-pong back and forth about the regular guy's view and experiences and the M.D.'s advice, knowledge, and analysis.

One thing that helps is regular exercise, and, as I'm sure you know, it doesn't have to be training for a triathlon. A modest amount of exercise that gets your heart rate up, on a steady basis, will do the trick. For me, this means riding my bike around our town rather than driving. Instead of doing my shopping at a grocery store a five-minute ride away, I shop at one of two stores, each a 17-minute ride, and cycle there at a brisk clip (and have a basket on my bike to hold the goods for the ride home). I also ride my bike to lunch dates. My wife walks a couple of miles each way to get coffee in the morning, catching up with her sis on the phone while she walks.

Or you may want to get back into traditional sports, like tennis or golf (but try walking and using a push-cart for your clubs rather than riding in an electric cart).

Swimming is terrific, as are hikes, and if your activity provides opportunities for social connection, all the better.

The important thing is to do something that gets you moving and prevents you from being mostly sedentary. Walk somewhere if you can. Use a standing desk instead of sitting. Every little measure you take counts — not just when you're working out on the treadmill at the gym.

The other thing that caught my attention in *Younger Next Year* is the importance of working on *proprioception,* which refers to your awareness of where your body and its individual parts are in space at any given moment. Proprioception often declines as we get older, leading to falls that cause broken bones, the possibility of extended hospital stays, and subsequent pneumonia or worse. The key to maintaining the balance and agility that good proprioception brings is working all the parts of your body routinely — not for strength, but for *nerve connection,* to teach your brain where your body parts are and to build fast, active connections and reflexes that will enable you to catch yourself if you happen to trip or knock into something. I remember being at our synagogue once when a woman walking toward the front tripped. I watched her go down in slow motion like a sack of bricks — and yet she wasn't able to get her arms out in time to break her fall. This is *not* what you want.

For me, working on proprioception means going to the gym twice a week, starting with stretching, doing a routine at each and every machine, then stretching again at the end. This is not about building my muscles but strengthening synaptic connections to my brain, and the whole effort takes less than an hour (when I don't run into people I know at the gym, which I often do — social connection as a bonus). Often, I bike the 4.5 miles to the gym to add some cardio.

That's exercise.

Eating also has a huge impact on your health. My wife and I have adhered to *The Zone* diet by Barry Sears for perhaps 25 years. The notion here is to balance *good* fats with *good* carbs and *good* protein in appropriate ratios and total quantities. The system is easy to learn and it's possible to follow it loosely, as I do, or stick with it more strictly, as my wife does. That kind of eating plan might not work for you; it can make sense to check with your doctor or even do a consultation with a nutritionist to get on the right track. But if you eat a wide variety of whole foods (and avoid processed foods), sticking mainly with plant-based options and good protein, you can't go wrong.

Now, do my wife and I always eat like this? No. Do we gorge on goodies at a restaurant from time to time? Sure.

But we try to eat healthfully most of the time. We let our bathroom scale be our guide: If either one of us has gained a couple of pounds, we're more careful until we're back at our ideal weight. If we find we've lost a couple of pounds, well, then we feast on junk. Just kidding on that one!

When we do go out, we try to ignore that oft-repeated command that many of us have heard as children: to eat everything on our plate. American restaurants tend to serve obscene (obese?) portions; often, a single restaurant meal fulfills the average person's target caloric intake for the entire day. Eat slowly enough to enjoy, and to notice when you're full. Then ask for a box and take the rest home. Most restaurant meals wind up being two meals — a bonus. Alternatively, we sometimes each order an appetizer and split an entrée. And if you're eating at home, be sure to serve yourself *much* smaller portions than a restaurant would.

Another thing we're able to do now, but that didn't work during our Long Careers, is to have our big meal earlier, in the 3:30 to 4:30 window. That way, we can work off the calories during the remainder of the day and avoid going to sleep on a full stomach. If we get hungry later, we have only a very small snack, just enough to take the edge off, around 7:30 or 8:00. Of course, when we have friends over or go out with them for dinner, we do so on their schedule and plan our day's eating accordingly (latish breakfast or very, very light lunch).

Whatever approach you choose, know that ***what you're really doing is delaying making your spouse or partner or children or closest relatives or friends become your caregiver.*** If you are in a partnership, know that deciding to focus on making healthy eating and activity an integral part of your life enables you to enjoy a richer and more rewarding life rather than declining by bits and degrees (or step functions) and having your day-to-day become less satisfying. You may even want to make a pact with your spouse or someone close to you and get at it, as my wife and I did quite some time ago. And remember that you'll get the outcome you want when you meet each other with mutual support, encouragement, and recognition, rather than by becoming the diet and exercise police. Each person has to *want* the good outcome, and the other person can only be supportive, but can't *cause* them to get there.

OK, one more thing that helps with health: attitude and self-view. An increasing amount of research shows that if you think you're old and incapable, you'll become that way! By contrast, if you think you are doing pretty well, have energy, and will continue to be able to do things and enjoy life, then that becomes the case! As Henry Ford said in *My Life and Work,* "Whether you think you can, or you think you can't — you're right." I once read a study that people who were shown subliminal messages on a screen (i.e., quickly enough that their mind picked up the message, though they weren't actually able to make out the words as one might when reading) that either said they were old, tired, and incompetent or that they were energetic, able, and thriving later found their actual level of energy and self-perception to be affected accordingly.

I suppose most of us don't have a way of doing this subliminal messaging for ourselves. But **we *can choose* to see ourselves as able, energetic people, still learning and growing,** and to have our loved ones support us in that view; and we can choose to embrace that view ourselves and to truly believe it. So, tell yourself that you CAN do things, that you DO have energy, that you ARE interested and interesting — because as my wife often teaches, language creates reality. As a result, you can help yourself be healthier, and you'll feel better and more capable for more of your lifetime. So team up with your spouse or S.O. or a friend and work together to have a positive self-view of your continuing capabilities in life, a bias toward learning and growth, and a helpful, positive attitude as well. (If this is of particular interest to you, check out *Mindset: The New Psychology of Success*, by Carol Dweck.)

After my wife, Carole, completed 17 years of teaching about interpersonal dynamics (think "relationships") at Stanford's Graduate School of Business, she had the opportunity to co-found a nonprofit to continue spreading her magic throughout Silicon Valley. We had many conversations about this, and in one, she said, "I don't know, maybe if I were younger, I could do this." At the time, I pointed out that she was 63 and had a dad and grandmother who lived into their mid-90s. Given that she was in *waaaay* better shape than either of them, she might well be around another 30 to 40 years! She was (and a few years later is) actually still quite young. And she did go ahead and co-found Leaders-in-Tech with the aim of changing the culture in Silicon Valley for the better. Still young! One just has to believe it and act that way to make it so.

• • •

CHAPTER ELEVEN

RE-CONTRACT WITH YOUR SPOUSE

Not cohabitation but consensus
constitutes marriage.

— Marcus Tullius Cicero,
Roman statesman,
lawyer, and scholar

f you're married or in a committed relationship, now's the time to decide on and invest in having a great rest of your life together!

There's a good chance you'll be together for the duration. If you've been married to your spouse for decades, the stats in the U.S. say you've got only a 1 percent likelihood of getting divorced after your Long Career (though that percentage is considerably higher if you've had multiple marriages or your current marriage has less than 10 years' tenure).

Of course, some people stay together because they're afraid of being alone, or out of inertia, their situation one of toleration rather than something better.

Instead of that, you've got an opportunity to **have a rewarding and enjoyable relationship.** And that won't happen by FM (f***ing magic, remember?). It happens when two people state an intention to get there, commit to getting there, and then work together on it. That's the re-contracting.

After those conversations and commitments, there's re-discovery. You're not the same people who got married back when. And you're not the same people who raised kids together, if you have kids. It's likely you're on new ground and will benefit from mapping a new course, which means figuring out what you still have in common and how you can support each other. If you're able to articulate what you'd like out of life going forward, that will be immensely helpful, too.

Knowing what you still have in common makes it easier to share activities, whether a sport or bridge or poker or travel or reading or entertaining friends, TV, movies, whatever. It may be that one of you is doing something to keep your business brain alive and the other is invested in volunteer work; either way, it pays to take an interest in what the other is doing and learn about what's going on for them, and then you can talk about it together. There's learning in it for both of you. Or it may be that you share a passion for something and you discover you can do it together, perhaps volunteering for the same organization, or going to orchid exhibits, or playing in a bocce league, like my parents-in-law did.

In my case, my wife and I like seeing our grown kids and our friends; we like travel, the arts, and entertaining; and we like to walk places together, among other things. My wife is also on her sixth career, and I enjoy hearing about what's going on, offering my two bits (if they're wanted — otherwise not), being supportive, and providing the life infrastructure that facilitates her career. I enjoy my Tapas Life, and my wife likes hearing about what I've been up to, providing *her* very helpful two bits when I seek them.

We've talked for many hours over a stretch of years about what we want out of this stage of life. For my wife, it's a career that does major good by helping leaders grow — very meaningful for her. For me, it's the flexibility and high interest quotient of my Tapas Life. I'm also intent on managing our finances in a way that makes life easy, with no nasty surprises. For both of us, we want to enjoy our kids (and our grandchild(ren) one day if we're lucky enough) and stay in good health to avoid one of us becoming a caregiver or spouseless any earlier than need be.

• • •

CHAPTER TWELVE

SPOUSAL CONVERSATIONS

Consider engaging your spouse with these conversation starters:

- What's your favorite way to spend an evening?
- What are things you worry about?
- What would make your life better?
- If you could have a do-over with me, what would it be?
- What was difficult when you were young? What was fun?

- What do you imagine I want going forward? What do *you* want?
- What changes have you experienced with your/my/our friendships?

Or pick some other conversation topics that are likely to get you two figuring out what you want your lives to be like going forward. You can go deeper with a book like *Connect: Building Exceptional Relationships with Family, Friends, and Colleagues* (Crown Books U.S. and Penguin Random House UK and beyond), by my wife, Carole Robin, and her colleague David Bradford. It's great!

Learning more about the "each other" of today will be very helpful. And you have a shared lifetime on which to build.

One person I interviewed, CR, noted the old joke that in retirement you can hang around the house as much as you want — you just can't go inside! In fact, he and his spouse are often at home together, in the same room, each with a book or on a computer, both very busy. My wife educated me when we moved in together decades ago: A couple doesn't always need to interact with one another; simply sharing space and doing parallel activities, with some regular meals together, can create feelings of connection, too.

When interviewing people for this book, I found couples who had fallen into a rhythm they liked, couples who hadn't taken the time to think about their rhythms but were worried there were issues that needed addressing (avoiders?), and couples who were well aware that there was work to do to strengthen their relationship. Not surprising.

Again, if you and your spouse decide to re-contract (remember: Discuss and decide where you want to get to, state an intention to get there, commit to getting there, and then work together on it), you can find life to be quite excellent indeed. As Robert Browning wrote in his poem "Rabbi Ben Ezra," it's likely you'll be telling each other:

> *Grow old along with me!*
> *The best is yet to be,*
> *The last of life, for which the first was made.*

By contrast, **if you don't *create* your new life together, you may well be leaving a lot of living and quality of life on the table**.

• • •

CHAPTER THIRTEEN

FAIL FREELY

The greatest glory in living lies not in never
falling, but in rising every time we fall.

— Ralph Waldo Emerson,
*American philosopher
and poet*

A ll your life you've likely done your best not to
fail at things. In school, you wanted to do well
to please your parents (or avoid their wrath) and
perhaps even because you enjoyed learning. You may well
have competed in sports or entered other competitions
(art, writing, music, etc.), and while you may have been
told that winning and losing didn't matter, as the years
went by, the competitive nature of life likely became more
obvious to you as adults and peers around you applauded

your wins and were awkward about your losses. It doesn't take much of this to realize we'd rather win than lose.

Once you're in your Long Career, you need to avoid regular failures if you want to be promoted, get more interesting work, and earn more money, perks, and benefits. Some managers are enlightened and realize that when someone fails, they may have been attempting a big and important pursuit, and that despite the failure, the learning is super valuable (and, therefore, so is that employee). But I have to say that I haven't met many who feel that way. For most, failing or doing poorly at things is career-limiting to varying degrees.

Failure can also mean getting stuck in a dead-end situation or being demoted or moved to a job or location you hate, or even being fired. And that can have a severe impact on your emotional well-being as well as the physical and mental well-being of your family.

No wonder most of us work hard from the beginning of school right through our Long Career, doing our best to avoid failure!

Yet once that Long Career is complete, *you don't have to prove a damned thing to anyone!* Perhaps for the first time since childhood, you can pick something that interests you and try it out — and you can be lousy at it! You can fail miserably if you'd like. It doesn't matter. All that matters is that you're interested, and that you try.

You're now at a stage of life where you can just be yourself. If you try something and discover you have zero talent for it even after giving it a good try, or it turns out you just don't like it after all, you get to mine the experience for the learning and the discovery of what future Tapas you may want to add to your plate. OK, I've said that a few times now, yet it's unusual and it can be hard for people to accept. So I've said it again. The cure for fearing failure is to try something with really low stakes and to enjoy the experience of either liking it or failing: both good outcomes!

A retired doctor I spoke with enjoyed mentoring young docs, so he figured maybe he would move even further back in the food chain — coaching college students on their med school applications. But delving into it, he found it was too much of the details of the application process and how to game the system and not enough human connection, so he shelved the effort in order to find something less nuts-and-bolts and more soulful.

I myself added a few Tapas to my life that were pretty good fails. After our youngest went to college, I decided to keep my business brain alive by working part-time in the solar energy industry. Since I had been in the semiconductor ("microchip" or microelectronics) industry for a long time, I knew something about the related solar photovoltaic technology. I created a custom résumé and emailed it to the CEOs of a half-dozen solar outfits in the area, eventually got through to a few, and was invited in by one for an interview. My offer to the company was 20 hours a week for *waaaaay* less than my earning rate when I completed my Long Career — a reasonable way, I figured, to try this venture out. We set it up as a try-buy: I'd do a few months of project work and we'd see where that took us. After a few months, I learned two things. First, I liked doing the projects but didn't like having to put together pretty reports. I'd been the recipient of those pretty reports, yet my own style when reporting on something was simply to share what I'd learned and discuss same. But I kept getting hit with, "So where's the executive summary? And how come there aren't any pretty graphs?" Which, to my mind, basically sucked. I also learned that half-time work was an unwelcome encroachment on the Tapas Life that I had been assembling. So, the solar idea and I parted ways. **A failure, with valuable lessons.** I learned that I was rather burnt out and bored with business, that an inflexible half-time activity was too much, and that I shouldn't try to be a fancy consulting type; also, my love of learning about new things was reinforced. This helped me be more focused on future Tapas selection.

My next idea was to teach Advanced Placement Environmental Studies (which the kids lovingly call "APES") to high school juniors and seniors and gear them up to help the environment (and perhaps influence the way they vote once they turn 18). I happen to be an environmentalist. After all, our kids and their kids need to live on this planet. Folks who can imagine any sort of life for their great-grandchildren in the hell that is Mars probably don't understand the facts. For now, Earth is all we've got for many, many, many generations to come.

So, anyway, I figured it would be interesting to teach APES, which I then discovered is considered part of the biology curriculum. I'd never taken biology, since I didn't want to pith/dissect a frog – yuck! (I did three years of chemistry instead, the last year consisting of running the chem lab and setting up experiments for teachers and their classes.) So I bought the Kaplan A.P. Biology workbook and learned biology. Then I studied up on all other areas of science covered in the tests that students applying to a teaching certificate program in Biology had to know. Then I took and passed the required tests. Then I applied to a graduate teaching program at a local university. They had me come in for an interview and take a written essay test to make sure I could communicate, which was easy. Then they told me I should find a science teacher in a local high school and ask to observe their class for 10 hours. I guess this was to see if I really knew what I was getting myself into. So I went to our local public high school, and the head of the science department said that to teach APES, I'd have to start out by teaching low-lane freshman Biology (because teachers are unionized and that class is at the bottom of the heap), and that's the class I went to observe. It was horrible: a bunch of kids who mostly didn't want to be there, many of whom behaved poorly (and this was the third- or fourth-highest-ranked high school in our state, out of almost 1,800). After one hour in class, I knew it wasn't for me. I mean, if I were allowed to teach APES, I suspected I'd be really good at it. But starting in the classroom I'd experienced, for an indeterminate number of years until I could move up the ziggurat to eventually be granted an APES classroom, was decidedly not for me.

All told, I had invested about four months in the process — learning biology, refreshing all of the sciences, taking three exams, doing an interview, filling out certificate program applications, chasing down college transcripts from 30 years into the deep past, and then observing a nightmarish classroom. A massive fail! On the bright side, I now know biology (though I suppose I did in fact know it well enough to have two kids…). I also came to realize that I'm pretty conversant in all things science-related. Oh, and that I could still communicate in English (truly, you get to be the judge of that).

The other silver lining is that nobody worked me over. My wife didn't count me as a failure. She and our kids found the whole process astonishing — they couldn't believe it when they saw me toiling over the two-inch-thick Kaplan A.P. Biology workbook. They thought it was great that I gave it a try, and when I described the classroom that had laid me low, they totally understood my reaction. Our friends marveled that I was willing to attempt such a thing. Nobody, absolutely nobody, told me I was a fool. Rather, they admired my effort. We were still able to pay our bills. There was no downside whatsoever. **OK to fail.**

Not that I gave up right away. I also tried private schools in the area, but one wanted teachers to also coach sports, not to mention be available for all sorts of things in the evening. In general, it seemed that they wanted me to give over my entire life to the school. Having a life already, that wasn't for me. One only taught A.P. Ecology, which was a little too academic and not applied enough for my purposes. So that was that.

Another retired doc I talked with started a medical imaging (specialized MRI) company with some friends and… they failed big at it. So he took the learning and applied it to a non-medical family biz and was able to grow it enormously. Try, fail, learn, apply the new knowledge.

Eventually, your path may take you to an outcome you consider significantly subpar. At that moment, you may find failing at something without suffering negative consequences to be an entirely new experience — and a rather liberating one at that.

• • •

CHAPTER FOURTEEN

BE FULLY

A journey never ends. Only the travelers end.

— José Saramago,
*Nobel Prize–winning
Portuguese author*

The decades of one's Long Career and raising a family are very much decades of *do-ing*. After these decades, you have the opportunity to focus more on how you are *be*-ing.

A couple of tools now in vogue to help you learn to *just be* are meditation and mindfulness. Simply put, these practices help you to become more fully present, to notice more of what's going on in the world around you and how you are reacting to it (both cognitively and emotionally) in real time. Do it often enough and you can learn to stop glossing over much of life and instead participate more deeply in it. Living more in the here and now can significantly reduce stress and anxiety. Think about it: If you're using energy to grind on what has already happened, rather than extracting what new wisdom you can and moving forward, you're wasting energy. Ditto with worrying about the future (other than creating a plan of action). In contrast, being present in the present maximizes the life you're living while reducing wasted energy and stress.

There's a good body of research that shows that if you meditate most days of the week, then within a few months, your brain's wiring will start to change in useful ways, and after a few years, you're on to a much more enjoyable and productive way of being/living. If you want to learn more about this, Jon Kabat-Zinn, developer of the now well-known Mindfulness-Based Stress Reduction program (MBSR), is a good place to start. One of his books is *Wherever You Go, There You Are: Mindfulness Meditation in Everyday Life.* He also has some good YouTube videos. You'll find this isn't about contemplating your belly button and saying "om" so much as it's about being focused and aware of what you've perhaps allowed to slide by unnoticed. A helpful step may be to try some of the many meditation apps available for free or a few bucks. It's easy enough to find one that works for you in a variety of situations. Headspace, Insight Timer, Happier, Simple Habit, and Calm are a few to consider. Monterey Bay Aquarium also has its great MeditOceans. That said, the best place to start with meditation and mindfulness is with a good teacher in a live experience (whether in person or online).

My wife is a fine example. She's been meditating every day for a several years now and is much calmer, much less of a worrier, much happier with how she is _be_-ing than before she started. She has several meditations she likes. One that starts her day is a gratitude meditation she does in the shower. Billions of people on the planet don't ever have a hot shower (or even access to sanitary water). So this meditation helps her focus on all the sensations and the context of the shower, and provides perspective on what a luxury it truly is. Something as mundane as a morning shower thus becomes a treat and a privilege, an opportunity for gratitude (which also brings health and happiness benefits) instead of being something to rush through on the way to getting dressed.

In chapter five, "Add Tapas and Stir," I noted that in my VIA survey, gratitude looms large. So one of my post–Long Career _be_-ing improvements has been to be sure to thank people and express appreciation whenever and wherever I can. This brings a happy moment to others and feels warmingly good to me. Lately, when someone is helpful and also cheerful, I thank them for their service and then note, "And thanks for your smile — that counts, too!" People light up, and I feel good about having spread a bit of joy. It's unfortunate that it rarely occurred to me to do this during the pressured days of my Long Career. Thankfully, I seem to have much more capacity for good deeds these days. Give it a try yourself — you might find yourself hooked, in the best of ways.

Another aspect of focusing on *be*-ing is *kindness*. A lot of people who meditate find they seek out more opportunities to be kind to others than in their past (per Luberto et al. in *Mindfulness*, and other such studies). Even if you don't opt to meditate, you may find that in your more spacious post–Long Career life, you have more capacity to be kind to others. And once you start showing a little more kindness, you become aware of even more opportunities to be kind and begin acting on those — and people are appreciative. It's one of those excellent upward spirals — what's not to like about that? Ultimately, you may find the world becoming kinder to you, too.

CR also feels he's being kinder to himself. He's certainly feeling more grateful. He told me that these days, he's constantly aware of "how fortunate" he is to have his spouse, family, friends, sister, and connections with people from throughout his life journey; he's always telling folks he loves them. He says "he's not the guy he was when he was working; he now has his health and no stress." He likes himself more and is comfy in his skin.

In this exchange from his book *Winnie the Pooh*, A. A. Milne states how fine it is to be fully present: "What day is it?" asked Pooh. "It's today," squeaked Piglet. "My favorite day," said Pooh.

Jim echoed the importance of "ensuring that I appreciate each day and enjoy it." Especially after his wife's death, he truly understands how fragile life can be.

Now let's get a little more philosophical. Perhaps you've heard of Maslow's Hierarchy of Needs, created by a psychologist named Abraham Maslow. It contains five stages of human motivation.[1]

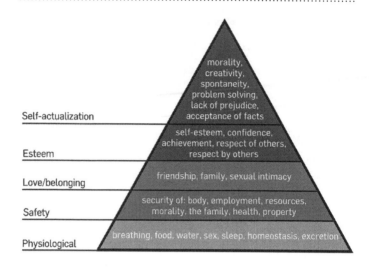

Maslow calls the first four stages "Deficit Needs," in that if we feel a deficit in any of these, it will make it difficult to move up to the next stage. But if you are able to overcome deficits that held you back in the first four stages, you'll rise to the top of Maslow's Hierarchy of Needs: Self-Actualization. In Army terms, this level is "*Be[*ing] All That You Can Be." **It's *be*-ing your best and most completely developed person.** This is the desire to do the best you can at whatever you're able to do. This is of course a very personal goal, one that is unique to each person. You have to know yourself well and understand a lot about how you rose through and mastered the previous four stages. And then you can stretch yourself beyond your erstwhile limits.

---

[1] Abraham Maslow's "Hierarchy of Needs" image sourced from Wikipedia

It's very likely that as a reader of this book, you've taken care of the foundational base of Physiological and Safety needs. Hopefully, you've been lucky enough to have a solid set of relationships that make up the Love/Belonging layer of the pyramid and will take this book's Social Connection chapter to heart going forward.

You may be blessed with plenty of the human (not dollar) wealth that comes from the Esteem layer that is near the top of the pyramid. Or you may not. It turns out that many of us have serious, and extremely valuable, work to do at this stage of life. Let's take a side trip to the book *Finding Meaning in the Second Half of Life: How to Finally, Really Grow Up,* in which author James Hollis makes the case that this "second half" is the time to revisit the circumstances and episodes of one's youth with the intent of freeing oneself from thoroughly outdated narratives.

You grew up with parents, and perhaps siblings, and the shifting nature of that household and the various personality dynamics caused you to adopt certain behaviors that "worked." Maybe they were in self-defense. Little folks are amazingly adaptable and figure out ways to get by in a wide variety of situations in order to survive to adulthood. Unfortunately, once we adopt those behaviors, we often carry them along over many years into situations where they aren't so very helpful, useful, or productive — and where they might even be significantly detrimental or limiting. What I like about Hollis is that he asks readers to go back and review what those early circumstances were and what behaviors we adopted — to look them in the eye, fess up as to which ones are not serving us well, and let them go. He asks us to reconsider who we are *today*, and which behaviors no longer fit either who we are or who we want to be.

ML says he "set emotion aside" when he was younger, and now finds that experiencing emotion has made his life fuller and at times more intense. His interaction with grandkids is the "purest," and he is "engaged most fully." He recommends working on one's ability to listen and process, and to generally be more aware. He fights the voices that say "can't" and listens to them less. He now lives in a "different frame of mind that is wonderful."

For many, there's real work to be done here, and it may not be easy. Some will no doubt shy away from it, but if you're willing to tackle it, you will find yourself liberated and much more complete as your own adult self. A therapist can be quite useful in such an effort. This is not a mental health matter; it's a personal-journey matter.

As an example, I offer my relationship with my brother when I was a child — about 60 years ago. He's six years older than I am (and was back then, too J). When I was small, he rubbed my nose in stuff I didn't know and understand, and that left me feeling stupid. It wasn't until my twenties that I realized that the reason I was so very ignorant was because I was in third grade and he was in ninth grade! For decades after that, I adopted the defensive behavior of jumping on anyone I suspected was vaguely implying I was less than intelligent, with assertions along the lines of "Yes, I know that — I'm not stupid!" You can easily imagine how jarring my response was and how out of place it felt to people who knew me and knew I wasn't stupid — especially when I said it in a very defensive way. Nothing useful about that! I kept up this behavior until I studied to become a coach at 59. Somehow, that training helped me wake up to what I was doing. I practiced smiling and saying, "Ah, good, thanks," whenever someone offered what felt like gratuitous advice, until, gradually, it came more naturally to me. Now, at 68, I can't say I've licked this 100 percent, but I'm a lot better than I was. And I like _be_-ing this way much better. Now my behavior is much more congruent with who I am, which is a more comfortable way to be, and easier for those around me. And I really don't miss going to that defensive place, which always felt bad in retrospect.

You could say I'm closer to the self-actualized stage — or at least more keenly aware of who I am and how I am. One sign you're there: You care less than ever before about how you're seen by others — you're responsible for and to yourself. As our kids would say, you give very few f***s.

Self-Actualization is a time of coming to grips with one's biases and prejudices (and, in my case, insecurities), releasing them, and getting more in tune with the world around us, as it really exists. Who knows — if you've always been a glass-half-empty person, this may be a time of life when you can come to see the glass as more than half full. And it's a time when introspection or conversation (whether you're an extrovert or an introvert) can help you see a more accurate picture of yourself. How does this relate to the Tapas Life? Well, a rising tide lifts all ships, and *being* more who you are — a self-actualized person — will make all Tapas and all of life a better experience for you and those you care about.

A fertile area you may choose in stretching yourself toward self-actualization could be a "flow" area, so let's talk about *that*.

You may well have found some activities that feel profound for you and that provide you with "flow." The concept of flow, put forth by Mihaly Csikszentmihalyi (he says to pronounce his last name as "Cheeks sent me high") in his book *Flow*, refers to the state we find ourselves in when we are doing something that is deeply engrossing — so much so that time flies and the rest of the world all but disappears. The activity uses a lot of *you*, but in a nourishing, not draining, way. It may not be *fun*, per se, but it feels highly satisfying or rewarding. It may in fact be downright difficult, yet when you look up after several hours, shocked to find that hours have passed, you realize you've experienced a very fine time indeed. Here's his model showing where *flow* exists:[2]

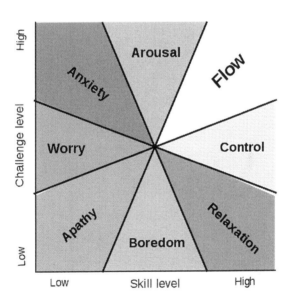

---

[2] Mihaly Csikszentmihalyi's "Flow" image sourced from Wikipedia

In essence, the top right corner of the chart notes that if you do something in which you have developed a lot of skill, and which is nevertheless very challenging for you, you will be in a *flow* state. You're using a ton of your capability, and reaching higher. It may be hard, but it's very satisfying. In the top left corner, you've got a big challenge for which you're very ill-equipped — that's anxiety! And so on.

For me, flow time occurs when I'm at the piano. I'm mostly a left-brain, logical guy. But at the piano, the music goes directly to my emotional core, bypassing the logical part of me in a way that little else does. When I start in on a difficult new piece, it's hard work and can even get frustrating. Yet it's common that I'll look up several hours later, completely unaware of the time, having experienced the effort as quite rewarding — a wonderful and uncommon way of *be*-ing.

If you have a flow activity, it may well have followed from chapter three, "Do Something You Love!" When I spoke with Michael, I observed that he has found flow in his photography, become phenomenally good at it, and deepened his self-knowledge in the process. To be sure, he's been enjoying photography most of his life, not just after his Long Career, so it's unsurprising that it provides him with flow.

Suzanne's undergraduate degree was in writing, with a concentration in poetry. But she turned away from that kind of creative expression during her Long Career in marketing and communications. Now, she has started writing for herself again, and says that often she sinks into a rhythm. She describes it as "stepping outside of time, as a kind of immortality" until the eventual need for food intrudes.

Like Suzanne and Michael, you may find your flow activities develop from pursuing a deeper engagement in something you're naturally skilled at and may have had in your life for a long time. If you don't yet have a flow activity, those are a couple of paths that can likely lead to one. And this may be the first time in your adult life that you have the time to explore and actually find one.

• • •

CHAPTER FIFTEEN

FUTURE TAPAS

The future starts today, not tomorrow.

— Pope John Paul II

Once you get started on a Tapas Life, you may find you've amassed too many desirable Tapas to sample them all at once. That's when you can either swap some out for others that feel more essential, or leave some to the side until it feels right to bring them to the fore.

I happen to have four Tapas that I'm holding off to the side (for now). The first two are volunteer work for EarthJustice and studying music theory.

EarthJustice is an organization of lawyers who sue state and federal governments to force them to comply with the nation's environmental laws. I'd like to help, but they don't have much in the way of volunteer slots. So I'm trying to see if I can talk them into a doubly Meaningful Tapa: namely, doing some coaching work for a few of their people (I've offered up to 10 pro bono hours/week). I call this doubly meaningful because I'd not only be helping another person get to where they want to be in life, but also helping improve the state of the planet for generations to come. Now that I have the CEO's business card, my plan is to give her a holler and see if I can make it happen. If not, I'll survey the landscape for another organization whose mission resonates with me and approach them about coaching some of their senior team. This is meaningful work I want to do, so I don't plan on giving up.

Music theory is also on the sidelines for now, though it's related to my time at the piano. As described, I love playing music written by others, mostly folks from the mid-1700s (like Bach) to the early 20th century (like Ravel, Gershwin, and Barber). But I would like to gain a better understanding of what these composers were up to. As it is, I merely learn the notes, then I interpret the feeling of the music (volume dynamics, speed, pauses, different types of key touch, phrasing, etc.). But I think it would be great if, after my piano teacher assigns me a new piece, I could analyze it before I start in on it, to make sense of it in a different way, before I play it. If you're into literature, you might compare it to the difference between reading a book and doing a "close reading" of a book. If you're a cook, it's the difference between following a recipe and knowing exactly why it works (like, what does baking powder or baking soda *do*, anyway?), as well as how you can successfully modify it.

I've been taking a music theory course online, somewhat in bursts and pauses. But I'm thinking about enrolling in a local community college and pursuing their several-year music degree (minus Psych 101 and such, since I don't need the actual *degree*). This would consist of music theory and appreciation (listening to and analyzing different composers' music), as well as composition (writing music). Hey, I'm 68, so investing a few years in something this pleasurable will have an ROI (return on investment) spread out over 20 to 25 years — well worth it! Once attuned to this Tapa, I enrolled in a continuing studies course at Stanford, nearby where I live, that teaches music theory through listening to great music and then unpacking bit by bit what the composer was doing. As always, once you key in on an area of interest, you start to notice people and opportunities that lead there, and so it was in this case. Thus, even though I'm not jumping into the full-up music degree for now, I'm still dabbling at this music theory Tapa from time to time.

Suzanne figures that in her late 60s, she has perhaps a five-year window in which to do things that require a fair amount of physical capability. And she's seen enough cases to have informed her opinion that "everything seems to hold together until 85, which is a tipping point."

Two other future Tapas are sitting out there on my horizon. One is the hope for little kids in my life. I find their whole demeanor and way of being incomparably interesting, and the way they learn and change week to week boggles my mind. They're a ton of fun and offer an excellent opportunity for supportive mentoring. I suppose it's because I most closely approximate a 10-year-old myself: unendingly curious and always fascinated by something new. Our 33-year-old son and his wife are expecting a baby soon, so with some luck, there will be healthy grandkids in my future. Of course, the only action I can take on this Tapa is to wait and hope. Meanwhile, my friend Ralph laughingly told me, "We love our grandkids, because they go home at night!"

ML wants to work on a narrative film based on his own screenplay. His wife, JL, sees life going forward as "wonderful." She's involved with grandkids and later plans some travel and gardening. She imagines that at some point, things will slow down.

MJ Elmore hopes to get deeper into music and songwriting eventually, and also some writing.

My other future Tapa is to try house-swapping — with our son. He and his then-fiancée mentioned that they intended to buy a condo in the big city, and that eventually they hoped to have kids and move to the 'burbs to raise them. So I offered up, one evening at dinner, that if they bought a condo that all four of us really liked — after all, they're really expensive! — then we could agree on an exchange in the future. When they're ready to move to the suburbs, we'll move to the big city. They could rent our house and we'd rent their condo at the respective market rates (which seems to be how the IRS would like to see it done). Looks like this will actually happen in a few months.

By that time, we'll be in the vicinity of 70, and we'll get the chance to repot ourselves in the big city (we are both city people). When we're old enough to be done with the big city, we'll figure out the next move, so to speak. In other words, it's the perfect real estate Tapa for the Tapas Life.

All of which brings to mind another thing to consider in terms of future Tapas, which is thinking of how you'll leave things for your kids when you die (yes, it will happen one day). To get ready for this kind of planning, you may want to sit with your kids and offer to answer questions they may have about you; you may share stories with them you haven't before; and of course, you want to be sure they know of possibly hereditary health issues in the family, if they don't already.

You may also want to start giving things to your kids, or, at least, earmarking them. You could ask each child whether there are certain objects around your home they'd like to have. If there's overlap, good to work that out now.

Ralph says, "Time is precious — you don't know when life will end." He gets a gold star for that observation, which leads to one last really, really important thing you may have already noticed about the future: Time keeps moving faster and faster. As my wife inevitably says every summer, "Is it September already?? Where did this year go??" In WWI, GIs, referring to cigarettes, would say, "Smoke 'em if you've got 'em." The version of that for you is **"Live 'em while you've got 'em!"**

• • •

CHAPTER SIXTEEN

CR'S STORY

This chapter is about a fellow named Charlie, whom I've referred to throughout as "CR" (since there's a different Charlie I've referred to throughout as Charlie). The two of us were on the board of our 1,500-family synagogue together, and over the years, he learned about my Tapas Life and was intrigued. So he built one of his own. I find it inspiring — and I think you will, too.

CR was an R&D manager at a tech company for around 40 years, and he pretty much liked the complexity of what he worked on and the people. Plus, being an action-oriented person, he appreciated that this was a Long Career where he could drive forward motion. In other words, he was good at it, and by and large, he loved it.

As it turned out, however, the company he worked for was spun out of a larger company as a stand-alone. Then, years later, it was bought by a different company with a very different management approach. After a couple of long years, CR, along with many others, was laid off. This marked the beginning of his path into the Tapas Life.

He hadn't been thinking about retiring, so other than his savings and investments, he didn't have a specific plan in place. He was afraid he wouldn't have enough to do, and this is a person who likes to be busy.

So he decided to catch up on his hands-on engineering skills, which he figured were rusty after years of being in management. Unexpectedly, right around that time, a volunteer opportunity that used many of the skills and capabilities he'd developed in his Long Career came up, and CR jumped in. He was happy for the chance to Keep His Business Brain Alive, as I recommend in chapter eight. At the same time, the organization he volunteered for is a nonprofit that does a lot of good for many people, so CR also felt he was doing Meaningful Work — Giving Something Back, as I talk about in chapter nine.

Of course, this volunteer work didn't instantly take up all of CR's time. He also took up biking to get and keep in better shape. And despite being an avid TV viewer, he decided to nix daytime TV in order to prevent too many hours sitting at home.

Biking, volunteer work, and walking the dog provided some structure, which prevented CR from falling into the untethered place. He also decided to go in with a friend and buy a small plane. CR had become a pilot in his teens but hadn't gotten the chance to fly on his own much during his Long Career. Now, he flies whenever he gets a chance, including a certain number of hours of instrument-only flying to keep up his "instrument rating." For CR, this checked off the Do Something You Love! box (discussed in chapter three).

Another Tapa of CR's is being a granddad. He told me a fun story about a granddaughter who visited. They went biking down the hill that CR lives on. When it came time to bike back up, the little girl protested that she needed help to get her bike back up the hill or, at worst, would need to walk the bike. In a teachable moment, CR patiently explained that she needed to ride back up the hill and was surely able. After the easy-to-imagine sulk, she did indeed bike on up the hill — and has subsequently become quite the strong biker and more self-confident to boot. So CR got to do a little mentoring, gaining the best kind of biking partner one could want.

CR's wife also loves the grandkids, which makes this an activity that fits in with how they see life together after CR's Long Career. CR's volunteer work also takes him out of town and out of the country, and he and his wife usually tack some travel on to these trips, experiencing other venues and visiting friends in far-flung places.

CR eventually expanded his volunteer involvement — first it was for his own faith community, but now he works with multiple groups across multiple faiths and secular communities as well. He tends to keep himself slightly overcommitted on this front, as he prefers not to have too much slack time. When it looks to him like there could be a dry spell ahead, CR is proactive about lining up "the next thing."

For social connection, CR relies on his wife and family, friends from our large synagogue, and others he has stayed in touch with over the years. These relationships keep him well nourished and are the sine qua non of a good life.

CR also experiences "flow" regularly, particularly when he is keeping his instrument-flying pilot rating up to date. To do this, he has to fly the plane without being able to see out the window. That means all available info has to come from his instruments, an experience he describes as "really hard." But he remembers saying, at the end of one four-hour session, that it "felt like 15 minutes." This is the essence of flow: It's a time that uses a lot of one's capability, is challenging, may or may not be *fun*, yet time flies right by (in this case, literally!) in a very satisfying way.

He also experiences flow when running meetings. This was true during his Long Career and is true now in his volunteer work. In both cases, this work is with sizable organizations and entails considerable responsibility. Helping diverse folks focus their efforts to move toward achieving their goals productively, once again, can be quite challenging. And yet, for CR, the hours put in can feel more like minutes.

Over lunch one day, CR and I got to talking about road trips. We agreed that the ones we like best have no agenda, no plan. Yes, we're aiming to get from here to there, but the route, the stops, the sights, the activities are all emergent, decided as we go. We exchanged notes about some terrific trips we'd each experienced, and what wonderful memories they've provided.

Looking forward, CR views life as something of an agendaless road trip in that he doesn't know what will be going on in his life five years from now. But he imagines it will be good, whatever Tapas end up on his plate. Because he is willing to keep sampling, keep choosing, keep pursuing.

I hope you're inspired by CR's story (and this book) to consider building a Tapas Life of your own!

• • •

CHAPTER SEVENTEEN

YOUR TAPAS LIFE!

A journey of a thousand miles
begins with a single step.

— Lao Tzu,
Chinese philosopher

Aimless road trips aside, you'll benefit greatly when you build a vision of what you want life to be for the next several decades.

Jim and his wife have a very broad view of what that means, and it's one you can't go wrong with: learning, appreciating, and enjoying together.

As you think about *your* vision for the future, do another scan of the topics in this book to use as a guideline. Talk about these things with your partner, family, and close friends. Be as open and honest as possible. Share your hopes and concerns. Experience the feelings that come with contemplating the years that lie ahead, both the slightly anxious and the excited. And use the checklist below to inspire and ground you:

Tapas Life Checklist: Things to Ask, to Do, to Plan

- ✓ What Structure will you add? Be sure you add enough so that you feel grounded rather than adrift.
- ✓ What's Something You Love that you finally have time for, whether you're good at it or not? What's a first step you can take to get at it? Take it!
- ✓ What will you Catch Up on? Remember, the sooner you deal with things that are long overdue, the more your life will be free of clutter, and the lighter you'll feel.
- ✓ What are some Tapas you might wish to add at some point? Build a shopping list of Tapas and look it over from time to time to sense whether this is the moment to pursue any particular one. Tapas you can engage in with others close to you may be especially tasty.
- ✓ Be attentive to and active about the Social Connection that is a cornerstone of health and happiness in the decades ahead. If you don't have

enough, find a way to add some. Little steps are OK for starters.

✓ Think about how you can make use of the knowledge and experience you've gained during your Long Career. Consider putting it to work doing something Meaningful — Giving Back. Absent this, you may well feel something's missing from your life.

✓ What you eat and how you exercise will have a *huge* impact on the quality of your life over the next 20 to 30 years. What Health commitments will you make with those close to you? I'm pretty sure nobody wishes to be a burden to dear ones.

✓ In what ways might you *Be* more fully? Reflect on whether you are still living based on mental models or scripts that no longer serve you — and whether you're ready to jettison them. How might you become a better person and like yourself even more? Take a moment to imagine your epitaph. What might it say? How do you feel about that? What would your ideal epitaph say? How must you *Be* more fully for that epitaph to be true?

✓ What are some things you might try at this stage of life that are longtime dreams of yours? Maybe you've not had the time. Maybe you've been afraid to try for fear of failing. Now you've got the time and you can Fail Freely with no or little consequence. Before you're dead, for goodness' sake, try a few things, just for kicks!!

✓ How and where will you experience Flow?

✓ What do you want your months and years to look like going forward? What will fill your life? What would an ideal day look like? What would a typical day look like? How would that make you feel? Write these reflections down. The more you can imagine your Tapas Life, the easier it will be to live it. And make sure you get your loved ones involved in the discussion. The more those close to you are in on it, the more support you'll have in getting and staying there.

✓ Consider reviewing this book from time to time, taking stock of where you are in assembling your Tapas Life. If you're given to writing, try journaling about your path forward. If you're given to talking with others, tell people close to you about where you are, sharing wins and learning experiences.

I wish you a happy and healthy, rich and rewarding Tapas Life. As for me, I see more piano (Flow), continued exercise (Health), coaching (Flow, Meaningful), cooking/wine, travel within the U.S. (already traveled a lot internationally), and perhaps grandkids. I see more social time with my wife as she gradually trims down her own work commitments, and more social connection with friends as they do the same.

Remember to *commit* to having some wonderful decades after your Long Career. And then you'll find that you can do it. You'll start seeing all the things along the way that result in a fine life for you — "the last of life, for which the first was made."

Enjoy!

Made in United States
Orlando, FL
20 November 2023